SpringerBriefs in Public Health

SpringerBriefs in Public Health present concise summaries of cutting-edge research and practical applications from across the entire field of public health, with contributions from medicine, bioethics, health economics, public policy, biostatistics, and sociology.

The focus of the series is to highlight current topics in public health of interest to a global audience, including health care policy; social determinants of health; health issues in developing countries; new research methods; chronic and infectious disease epidemics; and innovative health interventions.

Featuring compact volumes of 50 to 125 pages, the series covers a range of content from professional to academic. Possible volumes in the series may consist of timely reports of state-of-the art analytical techniques, reports from the field, snapshots of hot and/or emerging topics, elaborated theses, literature reviews, and in-depth case studies. Both solicited and unsolicited manuscripts are considered for publication in this series.

Briefs are published as part of Springer's eBook collection, with millions of users worldwide. In addition, Briefs are available for individual print and electronic purchase.

Briefs are characterized by fast, global electronic dissemination, standard publishing contracts, easy-to-use manuscript preparation and formatting guidelines, and expedited production schedules. We aim for publication 8–12 weeks after acceptance.

More information about this series at http://www.springer.com/series/10138

Monica M. Taylor

Rural Health Disparities

Public Health, Policy, and Planning
Approaches

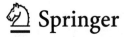 Springer

Monica M. Taylor
Faculty-Healthcare Administration
and Business
Colorado State University—Global Campus
Greenwood Village, CO, USA

Health Services Management
University of Maryland University College
Adelphi, MD, USA

ISSN 2192-3698 ISSN 2192-3701 (electronic)
SpringerBriefs in Public Health
ISBN 978-3-030-11466-4 ISBN 978-3-030-11467-1 (eBook)
https://doi.org/10.1007/978-3-030-11467-1

Library of Congress Control Number: 2019932718

This Springer imprint is published by the registered company Springer Nature Switzerland AG
The registered company address is: Gewerbestrasse 11, 6330 Cham, Switzerland

*To my dear mother, Patricia Ann and
my children, Christian, Chase and Taylor,
whose endless comedy is the joy of my life
(Psalm: 118:5)*

Contents

1 National and Global Rural Health Crisis: Spatial Injustice 1
  Heart Disease 4
  Unintentional Injuries 6
  Cancer 9
  Conclusion 12
  References 12

2 Environmental Injustices in Rural America 17
  Fracking Technology: Justice for Rural Areas or an Environmental
  Nightmare? 18
  References 23

3 Public Health Solutions to Rural Health Disparities 25
  Social Determinants of Health and Rural Populations 26
  SDH: Segregation in Rural Schools 26
  SDH: Toxic Exposure 28
  SDH: Food Insecurity 29
  SDH: Digital Technology 30
    Public Health Solutions 32
  References 33

4 Rural Health Disparities: The Policy Perspective 37
  Policy Approaches 39
    Policy Logic Model for Rural Communities 39
    Health in All Policies Approach for Rural Communities 44
  Concluding Remarks for Policy Models for Rural Health Disparities . . . 46
  References 47

5   Rural Health Disparities: The Planning Perspective   49
    Rural Planning   51
    Theory   52
    Approaches   53
    Concluding Remarks on Planning Goals for Rural Health
    Disparities   55
    References   55

6   Conclusion: A Progressive Vision   57

Index   59

Introduction

This book was purposed for academics, practitioners and students who have an inner passion to eradicate geographical health disparities. I wanted to impose theories and models for sustainable change using a multidisciplinary approach: public health, planning and public policy.

Admittedly, I interjected a few political paradigms throughout the book—a practice I found extremely hard to avoid when I am angered by poor health outcomes associated with marginalization, oppression, economic deprivation, segregation, social and environmental injustices and so on.

Nevertheless, rural health from a public health, planning and public policy lens remains central to the objectives of this book. While the need for a public health conversation relative to this book may appear elementary, seemingly enough, the approaches considered are grounded in international discourse on the significance of the social determinants of health. Although articulated differently, the themes remain the same. The cry for justice in the distribution of resources in rural communities is repetitive. Any other objective proposed by practitioners places sustainability at risk along with the uncertainty of health outcomes for rural populations.

The environmental injustice chapter highlights a different set of problems in rural communities. Certainly, I am aware this chapter falls under the auspices of public health. However, the environmental oppression rural communities endured in recent decades deserve its own spotlight and recognition of the extent of political and economic forces on geographical health disparities.

What to Expect

Chapter 1: summarizes the top causes of mortality for rural populations at both the global and national levels; Chap. 2: provides an example of environmental justice issues that threaten the rural landscape; Chap. 3: offers practitioners public health strategies to address rural health disparities; Chap. 4: provides theories and policy models for rural health disparities; Chap. 5: provides theoretical foundations and solutions for rural planners and Chap. 6: concludes with a vision for alleviating rural health disparities.

Chapter 1
National and Global Rural Health Crisis: Spatial Injustice

The scientific literature supplies indisputable evidence on health differences between populations based on race, ethnicity and socioeconomic status. However, studies centered on geographic health differences provide a more robust indicator on striking health disparities in morbidity, mortality and diminished quality of life. In the urban versus rural landscape, evidence of spatial injustices in health depicts the latter with an unequal burden of disease. Rural populations suffer disproportionately from disease prevalence across a range of ailments. Hence, the study of the epidemiology of disease and health disparities must yield stronger consideration to rurality. Variations in health status, behaviors and the distribution of resources are manifested when regional differences are emphasized.

Health disparities and rurality are compounded by economic deprivation and as some researchers would contend, race and ethnicity. The scientific literature tells us that we can not disregard the effects of race, however, geographical and economic factors exacerbate health differences within and between races. When research designs applied geographic indicators in racial and ethnic health outcomes, prominent differences were observed (Towne et al. 2017). For example, rural Whites and Blacks were less likely to report they were in good or excellent health compared to their urban counterparts. When researchers examined screening behaviors based geography and within race, whites in rural areas had fewer dental visits and blacks in rural locales had less cholesterol and cervical cancer screenings compared to their urban counterparts (Caldwell et al. 2016). When mortality rates were observed, blacks and whites who resided in rural areas were more susceptible to higher mortality (James and Cossman 2017). Overall, rurality contributed to higher mortality rates across all racial and ethnic groups (Singh and Siahpush 2014). Compared to their urban residents, mortality was 13% higher in rural whites, 8% higher in rural blacks, and 162% higher for rural American Indian/Alaskan Natives.

While an acknowledgement of race may bear some significance to health disparities, an emphasis on spatial patterns in the context of race substantiates the association. For example, disparities in mortality between and within blacks and whites were explored based on regions (James and Cossman 2017; Cossman et al. 2016). Prior to the 1980s, mortality trends reflected an urban mortality penalty, such that

© The Author(s), under exclusive license to Springer Nature Switzerland AG 2019
M. M. Taylor, *Rural Health Disparities*, SpringerBriefs in Public Health,
https://doi.org/10.1007/978-3-030-11467-1_1

people who lived in urban places with large population densities, died at higher rates due to infectious and contagious diseases relative to rural populations. Improvements in public health infrastructure prompted adequate sewage systems, water and food quality, and access to vaccinations. This ultimately increased life expectancy to 50% by the late 1940s for urban populations. Recent studies now show a reverse trend demonstrative of a rural mortality penalty. In the U.S., the rural mortality penalty, increased substantially in the past few decades. The white rural mortality penalty was more evident in the 1980s and the black rural mortality penalty manifested in the 1990s. Excess death rates showed greater distinction in the most rural regions in the U.S. for both races. Overall, death rates have improved for urban and rural blacks and whites albeit, such improvements occurred at a slower rate in rural populations. At an even greater disadvantage were blacks in rural areas, where the change in death rates lagged behind rural whites. Researchers attributed this to severe poverty. Today, the rural mortality penalty for both races are nearly compatible.

Health and social determinants for excess and increasing rural mortality were related to poverty, lifestyle, household composition, income inequality, inadequate access to hospitals and physicians and demographic changes (James 2014). An even greater mortality penalty exists in more rural regions in the South, densely populated by blacks who were systematically subjected to barriers to economic opportunities, intergenerational poverty, and additional social determinants of health including discrimination, segregation, access to healthcare and public health infrastructure. Consistent with the health disparities literature, areas with steeper poverty had diminished health outcomes, higher morbidity and mortality. Poorer blacks in rural areas were nearly three times more likely to die from all causes of death and prematurely compared to affluent blacks and whites in urban areas (Singh and Siahpush 2014). The death rate overall for populations in non-metropolitan areas exceeded metropolitan populations by 16% (Singh and Siahpush 2014). Premature deaths from all causes was 26% higher in non-metro areas. The causes of death which attributed to the increasing health gap between rural and urban areas included heart disease, unintentional injuries, cancer, COPD and pneumonia/influenza.

When chronic illnesses were assessed between race and ethnicity in rural areas, American Indian/Alaskan Native (AI/AN) (23.2%) showed higher rates of mental illness followed by whites (20.3%), Hispanics (15.9%), Blacks (15.8%) and Asians (5.8%) (James et al. 2017). Blacks had higher obesity rates (45.9%) compared to 38.5% in the AI/AN population and 15.8% among Asians. Severe obesity prevalence was higher among blacks (12%) in rural areas followed by AI/AN at 6.9% and Whites at 5%. In terms of health behaviors among rural racial and ethnic populations, fewer Hispanics (17%) and Asians smoked (10.9%) compared to non-hispanic whites (24.7%) and binge drinking was highest in Whites and AI/AN.

Researchers examined the extent of mortality disparities based on geography and gender within race and ethnicity (Singh and Siahpush 2014). Males and females in non-metropolitan areas demonstrated increasing risks for mortality, while urban residents showed diminishing mortality. The average rate of decline for all causes of mortality occurred faster for women in metropolitan areas compared to women in non-metropolitan areas at 0.98 and 0.68%, respectively between 1969 and 2009. A similar paradox occurred among men who lived in metropolitan and non-metropolitan areas during the same time period, with the former illustrating more rapid declines in mortality at 1.40% and the latter at 1.09% annually. When researchers examined geography and gender in the context of race, White and Black males and females in metropolitan and non-metropolitan areas showed comparable trends. Mortality was slower, annually, for non-metropolitan blacks, at 0.80% compared to blacks in metropolitan areas at 1.01%. Blacks in urban areas and American Indian/Alaska Native (AI/AN) men in rural areas had increasingly higher death rates. Among women, rural AI/AN women had higher death rates than their urban counterparts.

When disparities were evaluated according to income and geography, the widening gap in health was more prominent. The income inequality hypothesis (IIH), poverty, geography and health disparities demonstrated some relationship. High inequalities in income, which describes the extent of the gap between the rich and the poor, was associated with lower life expectancy, poorer health outcomes, a lack of social trust and diminished psychosocial capacity (Kragten and Rozer 2016). Between 1970 and 2010, disparities in death rates rose between affluent groups and low income populations concurrently with increasing income inequality in developed countries including the U.S. and United Kingdom (Truesdale and Jencks 2016). At the U.S. county level, high income inequality levels was more prevalent among metropolitan and non-metropolitan U.S. counties than ever before (PRB 2017). By 2014, over 1300 additional counties had both high poverty and higher income inequality levels. In 1989, only 29% of U.S. counties experienced high income inequality compared to 41% by 2014. In large metropolitan counties, high income inequality levels combined with poverty grew from 11% in 1989 to 21% by 2014 and in non-metropolitan areas, such levels grew from 35% in 1989 to 44% by 2014.

In the past four decades, the disparity gap increased between the urban rich and the rural poor for all causes of mortality, which was consistent with the IIH (Singh and Siahpush 2014). Between 1990 and 1992, mortality rates for poor rural residents was 25% higher than mortality rates for residents in affluent urban areas. By 2005–2009, the health disparity gap rose to 42%. In the same timeframe the rural poor was 4.7 times more likely to die from HIV/AIDS than affluent urban populations. Mortality rates for persons between the ages of 25–44 was three times higher and infant death rates was nearly twice as higher.

Irrespective of factors associated with race, gender, poverty, income inequality and rural health disparities described in this chapter, geographical inequities warrant a point of investigation on the extent of the problem to provide justification for feasible solutions. This chapter now turns to a review of a few of the major causes of deaths in the U.S. impacting rural America. While not exhaustive, a description of select diseases and health conditions is explained to illustrate salient differences in outcomes for both rural and urban residents and draws comparisons to health outcomes for rural populations in other countries.

From 1999 to 2014, research studies using the National Vital Statistics System, showed non-metropolitan residents experienced greater excess deaths from the five leading causes of mortality for the U.S. compared to metropolitan residents (Moy et al. 2017). These deaths could have potentially been avoided if public health infrastructure was available and implemented in underserved areas (Garcia et al. 2017). The five leading causes of death include heart disease, stroke, cancer, unintentional injury and chronic lower respiratory diseases (CLRD). Rural deaths occurred at a rate of 830.5 per 100,000 population compared to 704.3 per 100,000 urban deaths in 2014 for all causes. Overall, death rates declined for heart disease and cancer, however, these declines occurred at a slower rate in non-metropolitan areas, which in turn, widened the rural-urban gap in mortality (Moy et al. 2017; Garcia et al. 2017). Many factors unique to differences in the rural landscape accelerated mortality or fostered comorbidities for heart disease, stroke and CLRD. Behavioral factors, such as tobacco use, in particularly smoking cigarettes, is a primary contributor. Smoking prevalence is higher in rural areas, which further increases exposure to secondhand smoke and deaths from CLRD in this region. Rural populations are typically sicker than urban populations, therefore, physical inactivity is more pervasive in rural populations as a result of debilitating chronic conditions. Inadequate nutrition and obesity occurred more frequently in rural populations, which escalated diabetes rates and hypertension. Obesity levels increased synonymously with increasing rurality.

Heart Disease

Most troubling for non-metropolitan areas, were the unexpected excess deaths from heart disease at 42.6% for persons younger than 80 years old compared to 27.8% for metropolitan residents between 1999-2014 (Moy et al. 2017). In 2013, 600,000 deaths occurred annually from coronary heart disease (CHD) and is currently noted as the leading cause of death in the U.S. (Go et al. 2013). Deaths from CHD have recently declined overall, however this downturn varied according to urbanization levels. Research from Kulshreshtha et al. (2014) showed that coronary heart disease (CHD) was on the rise in rural areas by 2007. Earlier studies revealed urban areas experienced higher mortality from CHD. In fact, blacks who lived in the rural South had higher mortality from CHD than in urban areas. Coronary artery disease mortality was more prevalent among rural men and women compared to urban residents. Women in rural U.S. counties had a 20% greater mortality rate from coronary artery disease compared to their urban counterparts in small metropolitan areas, which had the lowest rates (Knudson et al. 2014). Men had higher death rates in all regions. Across all regions: In the Northeast, death rates were higher in inner cities, and in the South, rural counties had higher prevalence compared to lower rates observed in suburban southern counties. Inner city populations in the West died from CHD at a higher rate, while small rural counties in the West had the lowest rates.

Heart failure consumes more resources compared to other chronic disease and resulted in more disabling conditions and loss of productivity (Young et al. 2016). National expenditures for heart failure cost $30.7 billion annually with a lifetime cost of $109,541 per person, and is projected to increase by 2030 (Miller 2017). In rural areas, 30 day hospital readmissions were higher than their urban counterparts and the risk of death within one year of admission was greater (Young et al. 2016).

Researchers identified some determinants and behaviors between rural and urban populations that attributed to this disparity. In rural areas, distance to healthcare centers, physician shortages, a greater lack of adherence to healthy behaviors and lower self-efficacy for self management of heart failure worsened health outcomes for rural populations living with heart failure (Verdejo et al. 2015; Miller 2017).

Heart disease outcomes due to unhealthy behaviors were far worse in rural populations compared to urban populations (Knudson et al. 2014). Risk factors such as physical inactivity and obesity was more problematic in rural areas. Physical activity improves cardiovascular health, however, increasing rurality resulted in decreased physical activity among men and women in nonmetropolitan areas. Men and women in the most rural counties in the U.S. reported the highest levels of inactivity during leisure time compared to large metropolitan areas. The West was the exception, where inactivity rates among men were the highest in large metropolitan counties. Similar patterns were found when obesity rates were compared in both regions. The greater the rurality, the more likely residents self-reported obesity. Women in the rural South and men in the rural West self-reported higher obesity levels in contrast to their urban counterparts.

Depression was another critical risk factor for CHD, which elevated morbidity and mortality risk for heart disease in rural populations (Fink and Jacobs 2017). Research studies showed that older rural women had a greater risk for depression and less access to mental health services. Geographic isolation, food insecurity, physical inactivity and obesity complicated CHD in older rural women. Most alarming, 35.5% of older rural adults presented with depression from primary care visits and usually avoided discussions or assistance with this disorder. In South Carolina, women who lived in rural areas with less than a high school diploma were more likely to report symptoms of depression compared to women with at least a high school diploma. Higher education among rural women was associated with less anxiety and less symptoms of depression. Access to health education materials on CHD and depression could potentially prove effective in rural healthcare settings.

Globally, some countries demonstrated similar disparities in cardiovascular disease risk among their rural populations. In Australia, rural populations had 60% higher death rates from heart disease compared to urban populations (National Rural Health Alliance 2017). In addition, hospitalizations for heart attacks doubled their urban counterparts and was 90% higher for heart failure conditions. Similar to the U.S., persons living in remote rural locations had greater smoking and obesity prevalence. Food insecurity, a shortage of healthcare professionals, lower income and education further fostered susceptibility to heart disease for Australia's remote rural populations. In the rural counties of Italy, 1677 heart disease men were followed over the course of 50 years (Menotti et al. 2015). Approximately 29% were diagnosed with CHD within their lifetime. Comparable to other nations, the strongest predictors of CHD for this group included excess cigarette use, physical inactivity and inadequate eating habits. In India, middle class women had more risk factors for cardiovascular diseases, such as diabetes, hypertension, abdominal obesity and lower physical activity compared to women with a low socioeconomic status in urban and rural areas (Mohan et al. 2016).

In China, CHD outcomes differed from the aforementioned countries and varied within its rural communities (Tang et al. 2015). Rural areas with higher income residents experienced a greater lifetime risk of CHD compared to residents in lower income rural areas. Researchers attributed this to changes in prosperity. As prosperity increased in the rural areas in China, stroke risk also increased. Researchers claimed that these unhealthy behaviors occurred after rural developments brought income increases, which lead to more consumption of sugary foods and meats. Public health education on diet and exercise accounted for recent decreases in risk factors for higher income residents. However, in the rural southwest areas of China, having a low socioeconomic status and little education was associated with disparities in CHD incidence (Le et al. 2015).

Unintentional Injuries

Transportation, poisonings and falls were the top three causes for fatal unintentional injuries in rural areas (Temple 2017). In urban areas, poisonings ranked first for fatalities followed by transportation and falls. Fires and burns accounted for 9% fatalities in both regions. Deaths from high speed motor vehicle accidents contributed to the highest disparities in unintentional injuries between rural and urban counties in the U.S. (Garcia et al. 2017).

Between 1999 and 2014, mortality rates for unintentional injuries exceeded urban counties by 50%. Opioid misuse and deaths from overdose accounted for such injuries, especially in rural areas. Inadequate access to drug treatment facilities or healthcare facilities which specialized in advanced traumas resulted in delayed care and reduced survival rates from unintentional injuries among rural populations. Emergency Medical ambulatory services in rural U.S. counties had insufficient medical supplies to treat patients who overdosed from opioids at the scene of an emergency. Ambulatory services in rural areas often traveled at increased distances to treat emergent patients or to transport injured patients to distant treatment facilities. In addition, behavioral factors such as non seatbelt use, texting, alcoholism and speeding all contributed to unintentional injuries in rural communities (Temple 2017).

In 2015, only 19% of the population lived in rural areas, however, fatalities from crashes was relatively higher in urban areas (U.S. Census Bureau 2015). According to the National Center for Statistics and Analysis (2017), fatalities from traffic crashes was 48% in rural areas compared to 45%, urban areas in 2015. Less than 61% of rural pickup truck drivers killed in motor accidents were unrestrained and fatalities occurred in 50% of rural passenger vehicle occupants compared to 46% in urban passengers. Deaths at the scene from motor accidents was 61% among rural drivers compared to 33% urban drivers. Additional motor fatalities occurred from rollover crashes from rural and urban passenger vehicle occupants at 38 and 24%, respectively. In these type of crashes, 66% were unrestrained in non-metropolitan regions compared to 63% in metropolitan areas. Alcohol impairment accounted for

47% rural motor fatalities and 45% in urban motorists. Repeat offenders accounted for 53% of fatal crashes compared to 45% urban drivers. In contrast, pedestrians killed by motor accidents occurred at a higher rate in urban versus rural areas at 69 and 22%, respectively. Speeding fatalities at night was also higher in urban areas at 63% compared to 50% in rural areas. Overall, traffic fatalities from motor vehicles have decreased from the period of 2006 and 2015 in rural (28%) and urban (18%) communities. In the same period, fatalities from alcohol impairment decreased 34% in rural areas and 24% in urban areas.

Poisoning from opioid abuse significantly impacted disparities in unintentional injuries in rural versus urban areas (Palombi et al. 2018; Dunn et al. 2016). While opioid abuse rose in urban areas, the rate of abuse was even greater in rural areas. Rural residents were disproportionately affected by opioid overdoses. Medical and non-medical opioid users exceeded their urban counterparts. Researchers discovered recreation and physical pain fostered rural opioid abuse. In fact, rural residents were more likely to be white, to have injected or snorted opioids, and most likely to use opioids in their lifetime compared to urban residents. The role of the underfunded rural context exacerbated opioid abuse due to the lack of alternative treatment options to manage pain, such as acupuncture, physical therapy or pain management services (Prunuske et al. 2014). In addition, 52.75% of rural areas were identified as mental health professional shortage areas by the Health Resources and Services Administration (McFarling et al. 2011).

Prescription opioid abuse has been on the rise since 1999 (Cerda et al. 2017). By 2014, opioid abuse increased by 400% and hospital stays nearly doubled between 1993 and 2012 from opioid related use. The death rates from this substance far surpassed heroin and cocaine abuse. In the U.S., Australia and Canada, prescription opioid poisoning was usually concentrated in rural areas, however, the epidemic spread from rural to suburban and then to urban areas (Pulver et al. 2014; Rintoul et al. 2011). Between 2000 and 2015, 72% of rural counties in the U.S. reported an increase in opioid overdoses followed by small metropolitan areas (14%), suburban areas (11%) and urban areas (4%) (The Brookings Institution 2018). Researchers attributed ecological factors such as greater pharmacy density in the urban areas of California to opioid related hospital discharges (Cerda et al. 2017). These areas saw a 65% increase in hospital discharges from opioid poisoning, however, rural areas in California were unaffected by pharmacy density. Other factors included residents with lower incomes coupled with physical injuries in the workplace, which enhanced the need for prescription drugs and added to the escalation in hospital related discharges from opioid poisoning.

Another rather, alarming phenomenon which occurred as a result of the opioid epidemic in rural communities were the number of babies born with withdrawal symptoms from exposure to this substance in utero (Villapiano et al. 2017). Classified as neonatal abstinence syndrome (NAS), rural counties in the U.S. saw a substantial increase in NAS from 12.9% between 2003 and 2004 to 21.2% by 2013 compared to their urban counterparts.

Globally, 80% of victims from unintentional injuries, namely falls, were in low and middle income countries (LMICs) and falls accounted for *more* increases in unintentional injuries in the rural areas of LMICs (Shirin et al. 2017; Stewart-Williams et al. 2015; Zhang et al. 2017). Studies from the World Health Organization examined the prevalence of falls in adults age 50 and over in China, Ghana, India, Mexico, the Russian Federation and South Africa. Researchers found that across these six countries, women, adults with chronic conditions, mental health issues and adults who lived in rural areas had substantially greater rates of falls. Environmental conditions predisposed rural residents into fall related injuries such as unsafe walking areas and open street gutters. Research studies showed that 38.8% of rural adults over the age of 60 in India experienced higher rates of non-fatalities from falls (Cardona et al. 2008). Rural Bangladesh suffered disproportionately from disabling conditions resulting from non-fatal falls and 66% of elderly population experienced higher rates of fatal falls (Shirin et al. 2017). The majority of falls occurred in women and rural residents who were uneducated, unemployed, widowed or housewives. Having a formal education in the rural areas of Bangladesh reduced the non-fatal fall rate by 70%. Higher income status reduced the rate by 10% and widows were nearly twice as likely to have non-fatal falls compared to married persons. Men were more likely to experience falls outside of the home, women had incidents within the home environment and children experienced more falls outside of the home.

In Canada, over 14,000 deaths occurred annually from unintentional injuries and rural areas were disproportionately affected (Burrows et al. 2013). Unintentional injuries were more pronounced in men and women who lacked critical social determinants of health such as income, education, neighborhood deprivation and specific demographic features such as separation, divorced, or being single. Remote rural areas experienced rates of unintentional injuries that doubled large metropolitan areas. Mortality rates from vehicular accidents more than doubled the rate for rural areas compared to metropolitan areas. Additionally, deaths from injuries resulting from burns/fires or drowning increased in small urban and rural towns. However, in rural remote areas, mortality rates were more prominent from such causes. In contrast, while Canada and U.S. rural populations shared similar, excessive mortality rates from vehicular accidents, there were no distinct differences in rural-urban deaths from falls or poisoning in Canada.

Canadian researchers identified several reasons for higher death rates from injuries among their rural populations. Road conditions, including narrow roads, poor lighting and higher speed limits, non-use of restraints in vehicles or helmets for cyclists were considerable factors (Harlos et al. 1999; Kmet et al. 2003). Rural residents were more likely to drive while impaired from alcohol compared to urban residents who had access to public transportation. Similar to the U.S. long distances to healthcare facilities delayed emergent care for injury victims, specifically among adolescents (Jiang et al. 2007).

Cancer

Cancer mortality rates in nonmetropolitan counties exceeded metropolitan counties in the United States, albeit there was some variation by type of cancers (Henley et al. 2017). Nonmetropolitan areas had lower incidence of stomach, liver, bladder and thyroid cancer compared to their urban counterparts, however their incidence rates were higher for cancers of the breast, prostate, lung, colorectal and cervix. While overall cancer incidence for all cancer types for both men and women, was lower in nonmetropolitan areas, these populations (both men and women) experienced higher mortality. Cancer deaths have been on the decline between 2006 and 2015 in the U.S., however, declines occurred at a slower rate in nonmetropolitan areas. Higher death rates occurred in these counties from cancers of the lung, colon, rectum, prostate and cervix, oral cavity and pharynx. Deaths from these aforementioned cancers can be modified from certain risk behaviors that were more prevalent in rural counties including obesity, smoking, secondhand smoke exposure, physical inactivity and exposure to ultraviolet sun rays. For example, substantial increases in lung cancer mortality and degree of rurality was consistent with more prevalent high risk factors (Singh et al. 2011). Within race, rural blacks exceeded lung cancer death rates compared to their urban counterparts by 22%. More importantly, disparities in access to preventive screening services contributed significantly to rural mortality.

When race, ethnicity and rural-urban inequalities were examined for lung, colorectal, prostate, breast and cervical cancers, gradients of mortality was associated with income gradients (Singh et al. 2011). Between 2003 and 2007, county level cancer mortality data showed that excess deaths from lung, colorectal, prostate and cervical cancers was more prevalent in persons who experienced extreme deprivation. Rural populations demonstrated more economic hardship and studies showed the cancer mortality and socioeconomic gradient was more severe in these counties compared to urban counties. Cancer mortality was 8% higher in rural counties. Within each racial and ethnic groups, socioeconomic inequalities persisted, with the most deprived blacks demonstrating higher mortality. However, geography remained a prominent factor for greater mortality in *rural* whites and blacks given the higher unemployment levels, poverty and lower education levels in this region. In fact, when gender and the rural-urban continuum were assessed, the two most economically distressed men in rural areas had an 87 and 70% higher death rate from cancer compared to the most affluent men in urban areas at 19 and 21%, respectively.

The environmental context of the rural landscape compromised cancer care for rural residents (Charlton et al. 2015). Rural areas have persistently experienced a shortage of physicians, including a range of specialists that have been essential in cancer care. Oncologists, palliative specialists, social workers and mental health providers are critical to cancer patients and interdisciplinary approaches for treatment. Oncologists occupied only 3% of rural communities in the U.S. (ASCO 2014). Social workers and mental health providers were nearly absent in rural communities and rural cancer survivors experienced higher rates of depression and emotional distress (Charlton et al. 2015). In the absence of sufficient mental health care providers, end of life discussions were unavailable to rural cancer patients. The use of public insurance is ubiquitous in rural areas, however, physician reimbursement rates were historically lower (Decker 2012). As a result, physicians have been less inclined to accept new patients, which further reduced access to providers.

Some cancer treatments were not available to rural patients due to limited availability. Radiation oncologists and facilities were not prevalent in many rural areas, which required cancer patients to travel longer distances for radiotherapy. Overall, in remote rural areas, the average travel time to academic-based health institutions was nearly 97 min. With issues of extreme poverty, inadequate funding for public transportation, money for gas purchases or car ownership, these barriers continued to foster challenges to cancer treatment (Onega et al. 2008). In addition, there is a dearth in hospice based facilities accessible to Medicare beneficiaries, further restricting access to critical cancer treatment for rural residents.

Rural and urban populations differed on their perspectives on cancer outcomes (Befort et al. 2013). Rural populations had a propensity for fatalistic beliefs towards cancer prevention and survival relative to urban populations. Fatalism regarding cancer events was consistent with thoughts of pessimism or hopelessness that nothing can be done to reduce cancer risk, a lack of understanding on which cancer recommendations for prevention were effective or the perception that everything caused cancer. Studies showed rural residents more strongly subscribed to all three of the aforementioned fatalistic cancer beliefs compared to urban residents. These studies also affirmed that lower education levels corresponded with each fatalistic cancer beliefs in both populations. In addition, knowledge about cancer was most commonly retrieved through the internet. However, with rural America lagging behind on internet access, and were less likely to perceive this source of cancer prevention information as reliable. Rural residents often trusted only their physician as a primary information source. Rural residents who utilized the internet for cancer information demonstrated lower levels of fatalism on cancer prevention and survival. Given this, increased access to providers in rural areas and internet access can foster accurate and reliable information to rural residents. In the absence of such essential resources, fatalistic cancer beliefs served as a deterrent for routine cancer screenings. When race and ethnicity was evaluated in these studies, these demographic factors did not demonstrate consistency with fatalistic cancer beliefs.

Studies showed that prostate cancer was more prevalent and mortality was greater in African American men and these rates were even higher among African American men who lived in underserved rural areas in the Southeast (Hooper et al. 2017). With National health organizations such as the American Cancer Society and the American Urological Association endorsing recommendations for digital rectal exams and periodic bloodwork to test for prostate cancer (prostate-specific antigen) for early detection, research showed that African American men still consistently scored much lower on knowledge of symptoms, screenings and risk factors for prostate cancer relative to other races and ethnicities (Weinrich et al. 2004). More recently, Ogunsanya et al. (2017), research identified younger African American men in rural areas in professional programs had especially lower levels of knowledge on prostate cancer relative to their urban and suburban counterparts. Also, rural AA men who were highly educated demonstrated greater knowledge of prostate cancer recommendations. Hooper's et al. (2017) research recognized three distinctive barriers to prostate cancer screening among AA men in rural counties in the southeast. Congruent with prior studies, knowledge was a significant factor, their inability to communicate effectively with providers and inadequate health literacy were also barriers. Some AA men perceived their visits were too short or felt their physicians did not provide sufficient information on prostate screening to make informed decisions. Others were more proactive and brought questions to visits and found this more helpful. In a qualitative assessment on health literacy, rural AA men believed their physicians used complex medical terminology, which impacted their understanding on the need to engage in prostate screening. Level of education was also a significant factor in these recent research studies since more than half of the participants in the aforementioned study had only a few years of high school education. These findings indicate a consideration of programs on prostate health at the secondary and tertiary levels in the school system, especially in rural areas.

Rurality impacted adherence to breast cancer screening and treatment recommendations in the U.S. and globally (Leung et al. 2014). When urban and rural differences in breast cancer screening in women 40 years of age or older were assessed in developed countries (U.S., Canada, Korea, Croatia, Australia, Estonia, Lebanon and Northern Ireland), studies showed that women in urban areas were more likely to have had a mammogram in the past one to two years compared to women in rural areas. Rural women in the U.S., Canada and Australia were at an even greater disadvantage. More rural women in these regions reported that they had never engaged in early detection for mammography screening.

Similar patterns were seen in rural-urban differences in breast cancer treatment after initial diagnosis at a global scale. In Rwanda, oncologists were nearly scarce in rural areas and the option for radiotherapy was non-existent (O'neil et al. 2017). Women diagnosed with breast cancer in this region had access to chemotherapy and endocrine therapy treatment at Rwanda's first public cancer center. However, surgical procedures were not timely and was documented as the most missed procedure within one year of diagnosis. Comparably, in the rural areas of Poland, surgical treatment for breast cancer patients at distal locations from oncological centers was accessible (Kurylcio et al. 2014).

Studies performed in Ireland found some variation in cancer incidence in rural and urban residents (Sharp et al. 2014). There were no differences in colorectal cancer incidence and screening between rural and urban residents. Urban residents demonstrated greater risk of cancer incidence for non-melanoma and breast cancer. However, men in rural areas had a higher risk for prostate cancer. When socioeconomic status was evaluated in the context of geography, risk of cancers of the neck, lung, stomach and cervix was much higher in urban male and/or females.

Conclusion

This chapter summarized a few of the most common causes of mortality in rural and urban populations in the U.S. and the extent in which these diseases burden rural populations in the U.S. and Worldwide. This chapter also exposed critical barriers to health: lack of education, income and geography context, which fostered undesirable behavioral risk patterns in the top ten causes of death. In the absence of these significant resources, justice for residents in the rural landscape is compromised and a rural cultural pattern of non-compliance or adherence to healthier behaviors is perpetuated. This necessitates advanced and expedient solutions to resolve the inequities in incidence, morbidity and mortality that cultivate health disparities in rural communities.

References

American Society of Clinical Oncology. (2014). The state of cancer care in America, 2014: A report by the American Society of Clinical Oncology. *Journal of Oncology, 10,* 119–42.

Befort, C. A., Nazir, N., Engelman, K., & Choi, W. (2013). Fatalistic cancer beliefs and information sources among rural and urban adults in the United States. *Journal of Cancer Education: The Official Journal of the American Association for Cancer Education, 28*(3), 521–526. https://doi.org/10.1007/s13187-013-0496-7.

Burrows, S., Auger, N., Gamache, P., & Hamel, D. (2013). Leading causes of injury and suicide mortality in Canadian adults across the urban-rural continuum. *Public Health Reports, 128*(6), 443–453.

Caldwell, J., Ford, C., Wallace, S., Wang, M., & Takahashi, L. (2016). Intersection of living in a rural versus urban area and race/ethnicity in explaining access to health care in the United States. *American Journal of Public Health, 106*(8), 1463–1469.

Cardona, M., Joshi, R., Ivers, R. Q., Iyengar, S., Chow, C. K., Colman, S., et al. (2008). The burden of fatal and non-fatal injury in rural India. *Injury Prevention, 14,* 232–7.

Cerda, M., Gaidus, A., Ponicki, W., Gruenewald, P., Keyes, K., Martins, S., et al. (2017). Prescription opioid poisoning across urban and rural areas: Identifying vulnerable groups and geographic areas. *Addiction, 112*(1), 103–112. https://doi.org/10.1111/add.13543.

Charlton, M., Schlichting, J., Chioreso, C., Ward, M., & Vikas, P. (2015). *Challenges of rural cancer care in the United States* (p. 9). Practice and Policy: Oncology Journal.

Cossman, J., James, W., & Wolf, J. (2016). The differential effects of rural health care access on race-specific mortality. *Social Science Medicine-Population Health, 3,* 618–623.

Decker, S. L. (2012). In 2011 nearly one-third of physicians said they would not accept new Medicaid patients, but rising fees may help. *Health Affairs (Millwood), 31,* 1673–9.

Dunn, K., Barrett, F., Yepez-Laubach, C., Bigelow, G., Petrush, K., Berman, S., Sigmon, S., Fingerhood, M., & Bigelow, G. (2016). Opioid overdose experience, risk behaviors, and knowledge in drug users from a rural versus an urban setting. *Journal of Substance Abuse Treatment, 71,* 1–7. https://doi.org/10.1016/j.jsat.2016.08.006.

Fink, K., & Jacobs, S. (2017). Depression, heart disease knowledge, and risk in a sample of older, rural women. *Journal of Rural Mental Health, 41*(4), 248–262.

Garcia, M., Faul M., Massetti, G., Thomas, C., Hong, Y., Bauer, U., & Iademarco, M. (2017). Reducing potentially excess deaths from the five leading causes of death in the rural United States. *MMWR Surveillance Summary, 66*(SS-2), 1–7. http://dx.doi.org/10.15585/mmwr.ss6602a1.

Go, A. S., Mozaffarian, D., Roger, V. L., Benjamin, E. J., Berry, J. D., Borden, W. B., et al. (2013). Heart disease and stroke statistics—2013 update: A report from the American Heart Association. *Circulation, 127,* e6–e245.

Harlos, S., Warda, L., Buchan, N., Klassen, T. P., Koop, V. L., & Moffatt, M. E. (1999). Urban and rural patterns of bicycle helmet use: factors predicting usage. *Injury Prevention, 5,* 183–8.

Henley, S., Anderson, R., Thomas, C., Massetti, G., Peaker, B., & Richardson, L. (2017). Invasive cancer incidence, 2004–2013, and deaths, 2006–2015, in nonmetropolitan and metropolitan counties—United States. *MMWR, 66*(14), 1–13.

Hooper, G. L., Allen, R. S., Payne-Foster, P., & Oliver, J. S. (2017). A qualitative study to determine barriers for prostate cancer screening in rural African-American men. *Urologic Nursing, 37*(6), 285–291. https://doi.org/10.7257/1053-816X.2017.37.6.285.

James, C.V., Moonesinghe, R., Wilson-Frederick, S.M., Hall, J.E., Penman-Aguilar, A., & Bouye, K. (2017). Racial/ethnic health disparities among rural adults—United States, 2012–2015. *MMWR Surveillance Summaries, 66*(SS-23), 1–9. http://dx.doi.org/10.15585/mmwr.ss6623a1.

James, W., & Cossman, J. (2017). Long-term trends in black and white mortality in the rural United States: Evidence of a race-specific rural mortality penalty. *Journal of Rural Health, 33*(1), 21–31.

James, W. (2014). All rural places are not created equal: Revisiting the rural mortality penalty in the United States. *American Journal of Public Health, 104*(11), 2122–2129.

Jiang, X., Li, D., Boyce, W., & Pickett, W. (2007). Variations in injury among Canadian adolescents by urban-rural geographic status. *Chronic Diseases in Canada, 28,* 56–62.

Kmet, L., Brasher, P., & Macarthur, C. (2003). A small area study of motor vehicle crash fatalities in Alberta, Canada. *Accident Analysis & Prevention, 35,* 177–82.

Knudson, A., Meit, M., & Popat, S. (2014). *Rural-urban disparities in heart disease: Policy brief #1 from the 2014 update of the rural-urban chartbook.* Retrieved from: https://ruralhealth.und.edu/projects/health-reform-policy-research-center/pdf/rural-urban-disparities-in-heart-disease-oct-2014.pdf.

Kragten, N., & Rozer, J. (2016). The income inequality hypothesis revisited: Assessing the hypothesis using four methodological approaches. *Social Indicators Research, 131*(3), 1015–1033.

Kulshreshtha, A., Goyal, A., Dabhadkar, K., Veledar, E., & Vaccarino, V. (2014). Urban-rural differences in coronary heart disease mortality in the United States: 1999–2009. *Public Health Reports, 129*(1), 19–29.

Kurylcio, A., Majdan, A., Mielko, J., Skorzewska, M., Cisel, B., Gryta, A., et al. (2014). Preference for surgical treatment of breast cancer in women from rural and urban areas. *European Journal of Surgical Oncology, 40*(11), S78.

Le, C., Fang, Y., Linxiong, W., Shulan, Z., & Golden, A. (2015). Economic burden and cost determinants of coronary heart disease in rural southwest china: A multilevel analysis. *Public Health, 129*(1), 68–73.

Leung, J., McKenzie, S., Martin, J., & McLaughlin, D. (2014). Effect of rurality on screening for breast cancer: A systematic review and meta-analysis comparing mammography. *Rural and Remote Health, 14,* 2730.

McFarling, L., D'Angelo, M., Drain, M., Gibbs, D., & Olmsted, K. (2011). Stigma as a barrier to substance abuse and mental health treatment. *Mil Psychol, 23*(3), 1–5.

Menotti, A., Puddu, P., Maiani, G., & Catasta, G. (2015). Lifestyle behavior and lifetime incidence of heart diseases. *International Journal of Cardiology, 201,* 293–299.

Miller, R. (2017). Management of heart failure in a rural community. *Home Healthcare Now, 35*(8), 420–426.

Mohan, I., Gupta, R., Misra, A., Sharma, K., Agrawal, A., Vikram, N., et al. (2016). Disparities in prevalence of cardiometabolic risk factors in rural, urban-poor, and urban-middle class women in India. *PLoS ONE, 11*(2), e0149437. https://doi.org/10.1371/journal.pone.0149437.

Moy E, Garcia MC, Bastian B, et al. (2017). Leading causes of death in nonmetropolitan and metropolitan areas—United States, 1999–2014. *MMWR Surveillance Summaries, 66*(SS-1), 1–8. http://dx.doi.org/10.15585/mmwr.ss6601a1.

National Center for Statistics and Analysis. (2017, April). *Rural/urban comparison of traffic fatalities: 2015 data.* (Traffic Safety Facts. Report No. DOT HS 812 393). Washington, DC: National Highway Traffic Safety Administration.

National Rural Health Alliance, Ltd. (2017). *The disproportionate burden of heart disease in rural and remote Australia.* Retrieved from: http://ruralhealth.org.au/news/disproportionate-burden-heart-disease-rural-and-remote-australia-0.

Ogunsanya, M. E., Brown, C. M., Odedina, F. T., Barner, J. C., Adedipe, T. B., & Corbell, B. (2017). *American Journal of Men's Health, 11*(4), 1008–1018.

O'Neil, D., Keating, N., Dusengimana, J., Hategekimana, V., Umwizera, A., Mpunga, T., et al. (2017). Quality of breast cancer treatment at a rural cancer center in Rwanda. *Journal of Global Oncology, 4,* 1–11.

Onega, T., Duell, E. J., Shi, X., et al. (2008). Geographic access to cancer care in the U.S. *Cancer, 112,* 909–18.

Palombi, L. C., St Hill, C. A., Lipsky, M. S., Swanoski, M. T., & Lutfiyya, M. N. (2018). Review article: A scoping review of opioid misuse in the rural United States. *Annals of Epidemiology,* https://doi.org/10.1016/j.annepidem.2018.05.008.

Population Reference Bureau. (2017). *Poverty and inequality pervasive in two-fifths of U.S. counties.* Retrieved from: https://www.prb.org/poverty-and-inequality-us-counties/.

Prunuske, J., St Hill, C., Hager, K., Lemieux, A., Swanoski, M., & Lutfiyya, M. (2014). Opioid prescribing patterns for non-malignant chronic pain for rural versus non-rural US adults: a population-based study using 2010 NAMCS data. *BMC Health Services Research, 14,* 563.

Pulver, A., Davison, C., & Pickett, W. (2014). Recreational use of prescription medications among Canadian young people: identifying disparities. *Canadian Journal of Public Health, 105,* E121–6.

Rintoul, A. C., Dobbin, M. D., Drummer, O. H., & Ozanne-Smith, J. (2011). Increasing deaths involving oxycodone, Victoria, Australia, 2000–09. *Injury Prevention, 17,* 254–9.

Sharp, L., Donnelly, D., Hegarty, A., Carsin, A.-E., Deady, S., McCluskey, N., Gavin, A., & Comber, H. (2014). Risk of Several Cancers is Higher in Urban Areas after Adjusting for Socioeconomic Status. Results from a Two-Country Population-Based Study of 18 Common Cancers. *Journal of Urban Health : Bulletin of the New York Academy of Medicine, 91*(3), 510–525. http://doi.org/10.1007/s11524-013-9846-3

Shirin, W., Olakunle, A., Md. Kamran Ul, B., Salim, C., Al-Amin, B., & Adnan A., H. (2017). Epidemiology of fall injury in rural Bangladesh. *International Journal of Environmental Research and Public Health, 14*(8), 900 https://doi.org/10.3390/ijerph14080900.

Singh, G. K., & Siahpush, M. (2014). Widening rural-urban disparities in all-cause mortality and mortality from major causes of death in the USA, 1969–2009. *Journal of Urban Health: Bulletin of the New York Academy of Medicine, 91*(2), 272–292. https://doi.org/10.1007/s11524-013-9847-2.

Singh, G. K., Williams, S. D., Siahpush, M., & Mulhollen, A. (2011). Socioeconomic, rural-urban, and racial inequalities in US cancer mortality: Part I—All cancers and lung cancer and part II—Colorectal, prostate, breast, and cervical cancers. *Journal of Cancer Epidemiology, 2011,* 107497. https://doi.org/10.1155/2011/107497.

Stewart Williams, J., Kowal, P., Chatterji, S., Hestekin, H., O'Driscoll, T., Peltzer, K., et al. (2015). Prevalence, risk factors and disability associated with fall-related injury in older adults in low- and middle-income countries: Results from the WHO Study on global AGEing and adult health (SAGE). *BMC Medicine, 13,* 147. https://doi.org/10.1186/s12916-015-0390-8.

Tang, X., Laskowitz, D. T., He, L., Østbye, T., Bettger, J. P., Cao, Y., et al. (2015). Neighborhood socioeconomic status and the prevalence of stroke and coronary heart disease in rural China: a population-based study. *International Journal of Stroke : Official Journal of the International Stroke Society, 10*(3), 388–395. http://doi.org/10.1111/ijs.12343

Temple, K. (2017). *Rural unintentional injuries: They're not accidents—They're preventable. Rural Health Information Hub. The Rural Monitor.* Retrieved from: https://www.ruralhealthinfo.org/rural-monitor/unintentional-injuries/.

The Brookings Institution. (2018). *A nation in overdose peril: Pinpointing the most impacted communities and the local gaps in care*. Retrieved from: https://www.brookings.edu/research/pinpointing-opioid-in-most-impacted-communities/.

Towne, S. D., Probst, J. C., Hardin, J. W., Bell, B. A., & Glover, S. (2017). Health & access to care among working-age lower income adults in the Great Recession: Disparities across race and ethnicity and geospatial factors. *Social Science & Medicine, 182*, 30–44

Truesdale, B., & Jencks, C. (2016). The health effects of income inequality: Averages and disparities. *Annual Review of Public Health, 37*, 413–430.

United States Census Bureau. (2015). *Geography: 2010 census urban and rural classification and urban area criteria*. Retrieved from: https://www.census.gov/geo/reference/ua/urban-rural-2010.html.

Verdejo, H., Ferreccio, C., & Castro, P. (2015). Heart Failure in Rural Communities, Elsevier. *Heart failure clinics, 11*(4), 515–522.

Villapiano, N., Winkelman, T., Kozhimannil, K., Davis, M., & Patrick, S. (2017). *Rural and urban differences in neonatal abstinence syndrome and maternal opioid use, 2004–2013*.

Weinrich, S. P., Seger, R., Miller, B. L., Davis, C., Kim, S., Wheeler, C., et al. (2004). Knowledge of the limitations associated with prostate cancer screening among low-income men. *Cancer Nursing, 27*, 442–453.

Young, L., Barnason, S., & Kupzyk, K. (2016). Mechanism of engaging self-management behavior in rural heart failure patients. *Applied Nursing Research, 30*, 222–227.

Zhang, H., Wei, Feng., Han, M., Chen, J., Peng, S., & Du, Y. (2017). Risk factors for unintentional injuries among the rural elderly: A county-based cross-sectional survey. *Scientific reports*, p. 12533.

Chapter 2
Environmental Injustices in Rural America

Environmental justice exposes power imbalances between the manufacturers of environmental pollutants and the populations unfairly subjected to the health effects of (Brulle and Pellow 2006). Typically, the discourse on environmental justice movements centers on racial equity and low income populations who experienced unshared negative externalities caused by polluters (Guidry et al. 2014). Disadvantaged populations further endured this multigenerational exposure to toxic materials in the air and water, including pesticides, invoking a range of illnesses from chronic to acute diseases disproportionately situated in economically depressed communities and in places where migrants work. Arguments to secure protections for such vulnerable populations are centered on industries that fostered environmental marginalization, environmental inequities, diminishing civic engagement, and political disenfranchisement where the burden of proof of exposure to environmental hazards fell on the victims.

Exploring theories that expand our understanding of environmental justice is essential. One trajectory to perceive Environmental justice is through political ecology which explores the influence of political, economic and social perspectives on environmental conflicts (Holifield 2015). Much of the studies on political ecology burgeoned on injustices and the production of inequalities in urban settings, and evolved to other jurisdictions including climate justice and food justice.This chapter returns to the historic roots of this discipline, that is, the rural political ecology. Of specific scrutiny in the chapter is the spatiality of environmental injustices in the rural landscape, giving critical discernment to land degradation, toxic water, air pollutants as well as the geography of marginalization in the context of capital accumulation.

This chapter uses concepts in political ecology as an approach to environmental injustice. More specifically, this chapter chronicles the gas boom industry and the changes that occurred to the rural landscape as a result, including its culture, land use, and the health of rural populations.

© The Author(s), under exclusive license to Springer Nature Switzerland AG 2019   17
M. M. Taylor, *Rural Health Disparities*, SpringerBriefs in Public Health,
https://doi.org/10.1007/978-3-030-11467-1_2

Fracking Technology: Justice for Rural Areas or an Environmental Nightmare?

The U.S. relied on oil from foreign countries for years, therefore, natural energy sources were explored. The Marcellus shale, located in upstate New York, Pennsylvania and Ohio, was identified as an energy source of natural gas for the U.S. (Powers et al. 2015; Finkel and Law 2011; De Gouw et al. 2014). The undisputed benefit is the 45 year supply of recoverable natural gas for the U.S. and the ability to meet air quality regulations on common pollutants imposed by the federal government with natural gas sources. The use of natural gas resulted in reductions in carbon dioxide, emissions and sulfur dioxide, which in turn alleviates climate change. In order to extract the gas, the most practical and economic method required unconventional drilling on the shale rock, five million gallons of water, chemicals and solids (i.e. sand) to release natural gas. Most commonly known as fracking, by 2004, this unconventional drilling led to a multi-billion dollar industry for Pennsylvania. Additional states, landowners and various industries could potentially benefit economically from this unconventional drilling process. Currently, Pennsylvania has already attained self-sufficiency in supplying natural gas (Considine et al. 2011). As a result, the U.S. now boasts economic benefits, cleaner air and international competitiveness in the gas industry (Minh-Thong 2018; McGlade et al. 2013).

Rural areas were favored for fracking activity due to the substantial land required for drilling (Ogneva-Himmelberger and Huang 2015). Fracking has evolved to a global phenomenon with the following countries participating: China, Argentina, Algeria, Canada, Mexico, Australia, South Africa, Russia and Brazil (Cotton and Charnley-Parry 2018). Some countries, such as Scotland, Ireland and Germany, and states (New York and Maryland) have banned fracking. Moratoria in Australia blocked fracking due to the government's lack of trust of the oil and gas industries to protect communities from potential harm (Bomberg 2017). U.S. supporters for fracking commonly included younger men, landowners and social conservatives who were not typically distressed by any potential changes to the rural landscape (Cotton and Charnley-Parry 2018). In the U.S., those who opposed fracking had less knowledge about the process itself but greater awareness of the environmental impacts. From an international perspective, people in the UK supported fracking when they were given prior knowledge about the process and Europeans were more likely to inform the public on the costs and benefits compared to the U.S. (Whitmarsh et al. 2015; Cooper et al. 2016).

While productivity from drilling substantially increased in the past decade and future plans to capitalize on this effort in other states were underway, the rush to drill on shale rock continued in the absence of an evaluation of the health impact or an assessment of any potential environmental threats to populations within its boundaries (Fink and Law 2011). In order to assess any environmental effects, disclosure of chemicals used in fracking technology is needed, however, this was not initially mandated by the Environmental Protection Agency. State oversight of any water contaminated from fracking was minimal. In addition, states lacked sufficient water monitoring systems, therefore, spills were documented. Some of Pennsylvania's drilling companies had already been charged with illegal water withdrawals. Fracking technology could also potentially cause air and soil contamination, however, improper disposal of contaminants during drilling has been suspected. Few studies on the potential effects of fracking showed that 73% of the products contained elements that caused some immediate adverse health problems upon exposure and some delayed effects (Witter et al. 2011; Diamanti-Kandarakis et al. 2009). These health conditions included gastrointestinal and liver disease, cancers, respiratory, brain and harm to the nervous systems and adverse reproductive problems.

Fracking technology, its chemical additives and byproducts continued to raise concerns throughout the nation on threats to water safety (Chen and Carter 2017). Large volumes of water from wells in Pennsylvania and West Virginia were examined to identify the chemicals used in the process. The studies showed 96 inorganic compounds, 358 organic and 63 chemicals were unknown. One of the primary concerns was the toxic metal contaminants in the inorganic compounds which were known causes of harm to the central and peripheral nervous systems. In addition, the organic chemicals contained some level of toxicity, including carcinogens. However, with appropriate protocols, such chemicals could be extracted. Recent scientific literature noted unconventional drilling can prompt seismic events in the U.S., Canada and Poland, created exposure to air pollutants, light and noise pollution from drilling and increased vehicle traffic accidents (Ellsworth 2013; Skoumal et al. 2015; Souther et al. 2014; Graham et al. 2015). Busby and Mangano (2017) reported a 29% higher early infant mortality rate in heavily fracked counties. During the period of 2007–2010, excess risk of deaths resulted from substantial exposure to fracking in counties in PA (i.e. northeast counties) compared to 2003–2006, prior to fracking. The southwestern counties that were not exposed to fracking, demonstrated modest increases in early infant mortality. Researchers attributed early infant mortality in these northeast counties to the naturally occurring radioactive materials which contaminated the surface water, caused by fracking activity In addition, the northeast counties showed that numerous violations per birth was higher compared to the southwest counties in PA.

Residents of Pennsylvania with the greatest exposure to the drilling process perceived their health at risk (Powers et al. 2015). Residents of rural PA, namely Bradford County which had significant exposure to the drilling process, expressed their concerns to the Department of Environmental Protection Agency (DEPA) and local legislators of their fear of water contamination and wanted accountability and access to information to confirm the safety of their groundwater. Many felt their clean water was being replaced by industry profits. While threats to public health was vocalized, the discourse on fracking centered on well compensated employment opportunities. Some residents were able to obtain jobs locally as opposed to outside of the county while others claimed that these jobs were relegated to more skilled workers. Some claimed that small businesses, physician offices, car and hair salons benefited the most from an increase in consumers as a result of the drilling process, while others believed the industrial boom would eventually leave rural PA in a toxic state with dismantled industry jobs. Others had additional reservations about the unconventional gas drilling process associated with compensation. Compensation was given to landowners, which varied considerably, who granted permission to drill on their properties. Landowners expressed some uncertainty on whether or not the compensation they received was fair based on lack of documentation submitted to the DEPA on measurements of gas flow on various properties.

Unconventional gas drilling was associated with structural, social and psychological changes (Cotton and Charnley-Parry 2018). The aesthetics of the rural landscape diminished and threatened its wildlife. Rural residents had limited outdoor use. The influx on new labor caused a dearth in housing availability and prompted price and crime rate increases. This, in turn, led to a range of mental health conditions including stress, depression and substance abuse. In Bradford County, rural residents were devastated by structural changes unique to their rural landscapes. Rural residents also experienced depreciated agriculture and were forced to forgo farming practices after the development of fracking technology (Powers et al. 2015).

Fracking technology and its potential for environmental harm to the public and specific groups that bear the burden such effects, contextualizes this as an environmental injustice issue (Cotton 2017; Meng 2018). As a matter of justice, all persons should have the right to clean water and air quality, unpolluted soils, sustainable wildlife and landscapes and fracking disrupts these basic rights. Research studies showed that vulnerable groups were more exposed to environmental injustices associated with fracking in three states (Ogneva-Himmelberger and Huang 2015). In Pennsylvania, poorer persons and the elderly were susceptible, in West Virginia, the poor, elderly and persons with lower education and in Ohio, children had greater exposure.

The perception of fracking on the basis of *equity* situates the discourse on understanding what the benefits, rewards and harm are and if such are distributed evenly throughout communities (Meng 2018). Key stakeholders with arguments for or against this technology requires consideration, opportunities for engagement and at the very least, transparency. Transparency in fracking equity includes identification of the intent to use fracking technology, not overlooking its long term effects on the social environment (landscape, security, etc.) or the health of the populations directly impacted, and an assessment of the potential benefits or costs to building sustainable communities.

Meng (2018) approached fracking from the lens of spatial justice. Spatial justice provides the context for environmental and social justice arguments related to fracking. Spatial justice examines if environmental policies on fracking are equitable and sustainable and if they benefit most members in society and not just the relative (elite) few. To understand equity by fracking technology from a spatial justice lens examines land-use abuse, pollution, water contamination and any threats to the landscape on affected communities and social structures, such as community security, labor markets, education and stakeholder engagement. Through an understanding of spatial justice and fracking, concepts in environmental justice is planted, which describes how differential exposures to pollution poses a negative risk to certain (low income or racial and ethnic) populations who live near this activity and necessitates environmental monitoring. Environmental justice requires fair treatment, equity in decision-making, environmental protections, access to a healthy environment and embraces the precautionary principle.

Explored in three dimensions, environmental justice arguments contextualizes fracking as distributional, procedural and recognition (Clough 2018). Distributional environmental justice evaluates the extent in which vulnerable populations share a greater susceptibility to hazardous facilities in their communities and the burden of negative consequences associated with fracking. The scientific discourse is mixed on the distribution of fracking sites. In Pennsylvania, the shale rock resides, disproportionately in low income, rural areas where the population is mostly white. Texas, however, is more ethnically diverse, but part of the shale rock is housed in rural communities with high poverty levels and the other is in urban and suburban communities with low poverty rates. Johnston's et al. (2016) research placed injustices with water disposal wastes from fracking primarily in low income, rural communities of color in south Texas. Also, most studies focused on the distribution of wells, rather than infrastructure, that is, the pipeline and compressor engines required for fracking (Simonelli 2014). The EPA permits minimal standards and regulations on the quality of such structures if housed in remote areas, which impacts rural areas. Technologies used to reduce emissions for pollutants for decades were not required in these locations. Areas with fewer than 10 buildings for human occupancy and buildings less than four stories within a certain proximity of the pipeline was designated as a remote location by the EPA. In addition, concerns on the safety of compressor stations have heightened since explosions and fires occurred in these stations in West Windsor, NY and San Bruno, California (Kohut 2013).

Recognition and procedural environmental justice embraces concepts in participatory governance (Gustafson and Hertting 2016; Clough 2018). Recognition emphasizes that all stakeholders impacted by fracking practices be present in order for a fair procedure to occur. The stakeholders present should be recognized as credible actors and their thoughts and opinions not disparaged in lieu of other actors considered experts. The attitudes and approaches of stakeholders are regarded as inclusive. Procedural justice centers the discourse on stakeholder inclusion in decisions on where to place fracking sites. Procedural environmental justice is feasible with stakeholders in urban compared to rural areas. Rural farmers in Pennsylvania, for example, lacked the mobilized coalitions that were established in New York to block fracking. Rural farmers were less experienced in collective action strategies and organizing, politically. Neoliberalism, at its best, also impacted procedural justice (Malin 2014). Global competition, corporate domination of dairy products, left farmlands vulnerable to demise. The financial benefit farmers in rural counties in PA received was commonly used as a safety net to alleviate debt, transition from the dairy industry or to save or preserve their farmlands for their children leaving them no longer dependent on natural resources, but to the production of unconventional gas markets (Malin and DeMaster 2015). Outmigration, retired farmland, coupled with other issues at the heart of social justice, including poverty, unemployment and food insecurity affected Pennsylvania's farmlands leaving farmers with fewer options for economic viability, which in turn, constrained land-use choices for rural farmers to permit environmental risks. Farmers complained that Corporations lacked transparency, which further compromised procedural equity. Some had delays in receiving royalty checks. Also, rural farmers had meager negotiating power on their leases or control over when their land was accessed for fracking.

From a social justice standpoint, discourse on the motivation for unconventional drilling of natural gas emphasizes the role of the community, social rights, grassroots organizing and joint decision making on fracking sites selection and if pollution or health is compromised by fracking. Franking site selection and distance to community is critical. Studies showed that fracking selection sites greater than 3 miles from communities resulted in less public health harm. The long term effects of fracking technology on landscape and infrastructure is considered, impacts on education, public health, employment opportunities and industry regulations on fracking, all of which coalesces with environmental justice arguments.

The scientific literature is divided on the breadth of economic opportunities available in fracked communities. Some studies reported job growth of more than 139,000 jobs in 2010 (Considine et al. 2010, 2011). Contrary, other county-level studies showed modest job growth (Allcott and Keniston 2014; Brown 2014). In Colorado, Texas and Wyoming, Weber (2012) reported a 1.5% growth in employment between 1999 and 2007. Research from Wrenn et al. (2015) measured the effects of job growth on local labor and accounted for employee residence in Pennsylvania's counties. These studies showed counties with high levels of fracking technology demonstrated only modest increases in employment for local residents, but substantial increases in jobs for non residents who commuted or temporarily relocated to these areas. As for taxable income for local residents, in counties engaged in fracking, total income increased by 6% compared to the 8% decrease in non-fracked counties (Hardy and Kelsey 2015). However, income to local residents for royalties exceeded employment compensation in highly fracked counties, showing evidence that local residents benefited the least from such activity.

The oil and gas industry profits the greatest from fracking technology (Willow 2016; Brulle and Pellow 2006). Therefore, the popular rhetoric on unconventional gas production centers on financialization. These industries embrace a neoliberal theology, which embodies economic expansion and free markets while citizens argue for human health, political equality and a sustainable rural landscape. The economic injustices from the gas boom industry appears in the extent in which big businesses benefit from the (gas) production process relative to rural landowners. The ecological aspects of capitalism lie in the negative by products created from the (fracking) production process and its pursuit for wealth which lead to environmental degradation, meager political empowerment and public health concerns in the affected rural communities. Finally, environmental injustices as it relates to distributive justice, recognizes rural populations as unevenly affected by pollutants imposed by those in power.

The concepts alone embedded in the rural political ecology requires a myriad of disciplines to alleviate public health disparities in rural communities. The first discipline that follows in the next chapter, is the public health approach, followed by planning and policy theories to address a rather pervasive issue centered on rural health disparities.

References

Allcott, H., & Keniston, D. (2014). *Dutch disease or agglomeration? The local economic effects of natural resource booms in North America.* Working paper, New York University.

Bomberg, E. (2017). Shale we drill? Discourse dynamics in UK fracking debates. *Journal of Environmental Policy & Planning, 19*, 72–88.

Brown, J. P. (2014). Production of natural gas from shale in local economies: A resource blessing or curse? *Economic Review, Federal Reserve Bank of Kansas City, 99*(1), 119–147.

Brulle, R., & Pellow D. (2006). Environmental justice: Human health and environmental inequalities. *Annual Review of Public Health, 27*, 103–124.

Busby, C., & Mangano, J. (2017). There's a world going on underground—Infant mortality and fracking in Pennsylvania. *Journal of Environmental Protection, 8*(4), 381–393.

Chen, H., & Carter, K. (2017). Characterization of the chemicals used in hydraulic fracturing fluids for wells located in the Marcellus shale play. *Journal of Environmental Management, 200*, 312–324.

Clough, E. (2018). Environmental justice and fracking: A review. *Current Opinion in Environmental Science & Health, 2*, 14–18.

Considine, T. J. Watson, R., & Blumsack, S. (2010). *The economic impacts of the Pennsylvania Marcellus shale natural gas play: An update.* University Park: College of Earth and Mineral Sciences, Pennsylvania State University.

Considine, T. J. Watson, R., & Blumsack, S. (2011). *The Pennsylvania Marcellus natural gas industry: Status, economic impacts, and future potential.* University Park: Department of Energy, Environmental, and Mineral Economics, Pennsylvania State University.

Cooper, J., Stamford, L., & Azapagic, A. (2016). Shale gas: a review of the economic, environmental, and social sustainability. *Energy Technol, 4*, 772–792.

Cotton, M. (2017). Fair fracking? Ethics and environmental justice in United Kingdom shale gas policy and planning. *Local Environment, 22*(2), 185–202.

Cotton, M., & Charnley-Parry, I. (2018). Beyond opposition and acceptance: Examining public perceptions of the environmental and health impacts of unconventional oil and gas extraction. *Current Opinion in Environmental Science and Health, 3*, 8–13.

De Gouw, J. A., Parrish, D. D., Frost, G. J., & Trainer, M. (2014). Trainer reduced emissions of CO_2, NO_x, and SO_2 from U.S. power plants owing to switch from coal to natural gas with combined cycle technology. *Earth's Future, 2*, 75–82

Diamanti-Kandarakis, E., Bourguignon, J. P., Giudice, L. C., et al. (2009). Endocrine-disrupting chemicals: An Endocrine Society scientific statement. *Endocrine Reviews, 30*(4), 293–342.

Ellsworth, W. L. (2013). Injection-induced earthquakes. *Science, 341*, 142–149.

Finkel, M. L., & Law, A. (2011). The rush to drill for natural gas: A public health cautionary tale. *American Journal of Public Health, 101*(5), 784–785. https://doi.org/10.2105/AJPH.2010.300089.

Graham, J., Irving, J., Tang, X., Sellers, S., Crisp, J., Horwitz, D., et al. (2015). Increased traffic accident rates associated with shale gas drilling in Pennsylvania. *Accident Analysis and Prevention, 74*, 203–209.

Guidry, V. T., Lowman, A., Hall, D., Baron, D., & Wing, S. (2014). Challenges and benefits of conducting environmental justice research in a school setting. *New Solutions: A Journal of Environmental and Occupational Health Policy: NS, 24*(2), 153–170. https://doi.org/10.2190/NS.24.2.c.

Gustafson, P., & Hertting, N. (2016). Understanding participatory governance: An analysis of participants' motives for participation. *The American Review of Public Administration, 47*(5), 538–549.

Hardy, K., & Kelsey, T. (2015). Local income related to marcellus shale activity in Pennsylvania. *Community Development, 46*(4), 329–340.

Holifield, R. (2015). Environmental justice and political ecology. In T. Perrault, G. Bridge, & J. McCarthy (Eds.), *The Routledge handbook of political ecology* (pp. 585–597). Florence, Kentucky, Taylor & Francis Group LLC

Johnston, J. E., Werder, E., & Sebastian, D. (2016). Wastewater disposal wells, fracking, and environmental injustice in Southern Texas. *American Journal of Public Health, 106,* 550–556.

Kohut, J. (2013, May 16). Fire, possible explosion at Susquehanna gas compressor station thought to be accidental. *The Times-Tribune.com.*

McGlade, C., Speirs, J., & Sorrell, S. (2013). Unconventional gas—A review of regional and global resource estimates. *Energy, 55*(15), 571–584.

Malin, S. (2014). There's no real choice but to sign: neoliberalization and normalization of hydraulic fracturing on Pennsylvania farmland. *Journal of Environmental Studies and Sciences, Springer; Association of Environmental Studies and Sciences, 4*(1), 17–27.

Malin, S., & DeMaster, K. (2015). A devil's bargain: Rural environmental injustices and hydraulic fracturing on Pennsylvania's farms. *Journal of Rural Studies, 47,* 278–290.

Meng, Q. (2018). Fracking equity: A spatial justice analysis prototype. *Land Use Policy, 70,* 10–15.

Minh-Thong, L. (2018). An assessment of the potential for the development of the shale gas industry in countries outside of North America. *Heliyon, 4*(2), e00516. https://doi.org/10.1016/j.heliyon.2018.e00516.

Ogneva-Himmelberger, Y., & Huang, L. (2015). Spatial distribution of unconventional gas well and human populations in the Marcellus shale in the United States: Vulnerability analysis. *Applied Geography, 60,* 165–174.

Powers, M., Saberi, P., Pepino, R., Strupp, E., Bugos, E., & Cannuscio, C. (2015). Popular epidemiology and 'fracking': Citizens' concerns regarding the economic, environmental, health and social impacts of unconventional natural gas drilling operations. *Journal of Community Health, 40*(3), 534–541. https://doi.org/10.1007/s10900-014-9968-x.

Simonelli, J. (2014). Home rule and natural gas development in New York: civil fracking rights. *Journal of Political Ecology, 21,* 258–278.

Skoumal, R., Brudzinski, M., & Currie, B. (2015). Earthquakes induced by hydraulic fracturing in Poland township, Ohio Bull. *Seismological Society of America, 105,* 189–197.

Souther, S., Tingley, M. W., Popescu, V. D., Hayman, D. T. S., Ryan, M. E., Graves, T. A., et al. (2014). Biotic impacts of energy development from shale: Research priorities and knowledge gaps. *Frontiers in Ecology and the Environment, 12,* 330–338.

Weber, J. G. (2012). The effects of a natural gas boom on employment and income in Colorado, Texas, and Wyoming. *Energy Economics, 34*(5), 1580–1588.

Willow, A. (2016). Wells and well-being: neoliberalism and holistic sustainability in the shale energy debate. *Local Environment, 21*(6), 768–788. https://doi.org/10.1080/13549839.2015.1017808.

Witter, R., Stinson, K., Sackett, H., et al. (2011). *Potential exposure-related human health effects of oil and gas development: A literature review.* Retrieved from: http://docs.nrdc.org/health/files/hea_08091702c.pdf. Accessed January 26, 2011.

Whitmarsh, L., Nash, N., Upham, P., Lloyd, A., Verdon, J. P., & Kendall, J.-M. (2015). UK public perceptions of shale gas hydraulic fracturing: The role of audience, message and contextual factors on risk perceptions and policy support. *Applied Energy, 160,* 419–430.

Wrenn, D. H., Kelsey, T. W., & Jaenicke, E. C. (2015). Resident vs. nonresident employment associated with Marcellus Shale development. *Agricultural and Resource Economics Review, 44*(2), 1–19.

Chapter 3
Public Health Solutions to Rural Health Disparities

The disparities in morbidity and mortality in rural populations are daunting to state the least. As such, this chapter proposes solutions for public health practitioners to consider as strategies to eliminate rural health disparities with increased attention on the Social Determinants of Health (SDH). Much of the prior and to some degree, the current literature rests on the doctrine of behavioral theories to change individual health related behaviors, which proved to have a modest, albeit, non-sustainable impact on widening health disparities, overall.

This chapter undergirds the SDH as a foundation for the development of critical public health interventions that can alter the life trajectory of rural America. The Social Determinants of Health (SDH) are the material resources that contribute to greater life expectancy and well-being for individuals in spaces where people live, work, play and age (World Health Organization [WHO] 2008; United States Department of Health and Human Services 2018). The availability of the SDH is determined by politics, social policies, which inform the distribution of the SDH at the local, national and global levels. The SDH is defined by the CDC and WHO includes income, quality education and job training, housing, clean water, sanitation, employment, universal health care, social exclusion, transportation, crime and violence exposure, discrimination, segregation, language/literacy, access to emerging technology, culture, food security and access to recreational activities. The Centers for Disease Control and Prevention (2014) further added physical determinants which include the built environment (roads, sidewalks and bike lanes), and environmental conditions.

Establishing equity in the SDH in communities at the onset of life, that is, early childhood development, influences increased life expectancy, optimal health outcomes, social, emotional and mental health. Investments in the SDH, especially during early childhood development, minimizes negative generational externalities that have long term effects on brain development and life experiences in children.

M. M. Taylor, *Rural Health Disparities*, SpringerBriefs in Public Health,
https://doi.org/10.1007/978-3-030-11467-1_3

Social Determinants of Health and Rural Populations

Rural populations face unique barriers in accessing the healthcare system compared to other populations as a result of geographic limitations (Rural Health Information Hub 2018; Heflin and Miller 2011). Rural areas experience a shortage of resources which consequently limits the scope and quality of the SDH. Inadequate transportation and housing and access to healthy foods are challenging. Compounded with these inequities, rural residents are disproportionately poor, which impacts food security. Disposal of hazardous wastes are problematic in these areas, especially in remote locations, which in turn, places their health and environmental safety at greater risk. There is a scant supply of human services programs in rural communities to adequately service the needs of the elderly and veterans. There is a shortage of resources to accommodate follow up care from hospitalizations and to address language barriers or cultural issues. Given this, the demand for human services is greater in rural populations compared to non-rural areas and therefore strategies to address a dearth in the SDH for rural populations warrants more exclusive public health interventions.

The remaining parts of this chapter identifies the extent in which geographical needs significantly impedes access to select SDH which further aggravates rural health disparities. An exhaustive list of rural social determinants will not be presented here. For example, typologies that exist in rural America, which include poverty, low education attainment, low employment or population loss is discussed elsewhere in the book entitled, *"Application of the Political Economy to Rural Health Disparities"* (Taylor 2018). This chapter highlights only a few: the impact of segregation, toxic exposures, food insecurity and digital technology has on healthy lifestyles for rural populations.

SDH: Segregation in Rural Schools

Southern Jim Crow laws were abolished in 1964 as a result of the Civil Rights Act, however, a resurgence of alternative modes of Jim Crow occurred in the 20th century in the areas of education zoning, workplace, housing discriminatory practices, racial zoning and conservative laws which restricted pathways to citizenship or goods and services (Highsmith and Erikson 2015; Kuczewski 2016). The dissimilarity index is widely used to measure the degree of segregation (Allen et al. 2015). The dissimilarity index measures the extent in which a particular social construct diverges from evenness but not systematic segregation per se. For example, researchers used the dissimilarity index to assess the underlying causes for higher occupancy of a racial group in one residential area compared to others or the presence of one gender in an occupation compared to another in the same occupation or the uneven distribution of low income children (or racial group) in one school district compared to others. Of interest to this chapter is the latter, with regard to income and rural geography. Segregation in America's school systems still persists through discriminatory education policies, however, decision-makers blamed private housing discrimination practice for the inevitable segregation in schools.

The discourse on segregation in American schools has mostly focused on racial composition in metropolitan areas, although geographical differences in education quality also warranted specific attention (Logan and Burdick-Will 2017). The dissimilarity index was used to measured poverty status of students, race and reading and math performance. Schools in rural areas share similar characteristics as schools in urban areas, however both are more disadvantaged compared to suburban schools. Suburban schools had higher test scores in reading and math and urban and rural schools performed nearly the same or had lower scores. Suburban areas with these school patterns have a large white population, however, rural areas are predominantly white and have higher poverty levels. Urban and rural areas have a higher share of students who qualified for free or reduced lunches at 63 and 58%, respectively. Black and Asian students were at a disadvantage if they attend schools in urban areas, whereas, Native Americans are burdened by the rural school disadvantage. White students had the highest poverty rates in rural schools, Blacks and Hispanics had higher poverty rates in both rural and urban schools, however the rate was slightly higher for Hispanic students who attended urban schools.

City schools have larger visibility and received greater attention relative to rural school districts. Rural school districts shared similar characteristics to urban locales and both deserved the same political attention. The special challenge of population loss in rural areas constrained the school system's ability to recruit teachers and provide specialized classes, particularly for elementary school children. Urban districts had alternative school options that included transporting children to charter schools, however, this opportunity was not available to rural students. The job prospects for rural student success was considered relatively low compared to urban students. Nevertheless, the implementation of education policies that permitted additional school attendance options was not equally recognized or applied in both locales.

Essentially, the scientific literature showed that Native Americans, Blacks and Hispanic students in urban and rural areas were at a disadvantage in their attendance of underperforming schools in the public school systems in America. The research also showed that these racial and ethnic students were equally burdened by concentrated poverty. Although rural school districts were predominantly white, these students were also disproportionately poor compared to their urban and suburban counterparts. This evidence showed that racial segregation in America's public schools, while relevant, the more prominent factor is economic inequality in education (The Brookings Institution 2018). The socio-economic status of student education achievement has far exceeded the gap in racial achievement and these changes were attributed to the Supreme Court policy in 2007 which ruled against race based policies as a proxy for admittance into K–12 public schools (Greenhouse 2007). Today, half of America's children reside in high poverty school districts as a result of the rise in income based segregation in public schools (EdBuild 2018). Bordering wealthy school districts in high income communities have higher quality schools with access to more resources, typically invested through property taxes. Economically distressed communities lacked both opportunities and resources to invest in their public schools districts. Communities that experienced long term poverty had poorer quality schools and lacked political power (Solari 2012).

SDH: Toxic Exposure

The built environment impacts life expectancy for rural populations. For example, hazardous road conditions are pervasive in rural communities. Rural residents drive at higher speeds compared to urban and suburban populations which led to higher rates of mortality from car accidents (Institute of Medicine 2006). Automobile accidents and traffic congestion in rural areas produced air pollution. Toxic exposure in the rural environment also impacted life expectancy. The World Health Organization (2018) identified chemicals, environmental degradation, inadequate sanitation, safe water, radioactivity, healthcare and industrial wastes as toxic exposures causing harm to rural communities.

The Federal government historically regulated the chemical industry in an effort to reduce possible environmental exposures, however, chemical releases have occurred with some being hazardous to the public's health and others being less detrimental (Young 2015). These unexpected, hazardous chemical events occurred during storage and use in urban areas or through transit related incidents, common to rural areas. The majority of these events occurred in Colorado, North Carolina and Wisconsin. In fact, rural counties in the U.S. experienced five times as many unforeseen chemical transport events than fixed facilities events. While urban counties experienced more releases, these areas had access to healthcare facilities for potential treatment for symptoms compared to rural and remote areas. In addition, studies from Gochfield and Burger (2011) found that rural areas experienced more dust pollution and pesticide exposure and indeterminate water quality (Gochfield and Burger 2011). Rural locations were often near agricultural waste sites which placed them at risk for exposure to animal excretions and mining materials, including arsenic or swine facilities. Soil contamination occurred from homegrown livestock and produce. Other studies found that air quality improved with increasing rurality (Strosnider et al. 2017).

Another source of toxic exposure in rural communities was discovered in the hog industry (Nicole 2013; Kelly-Reif and Wing 2016; Wing 2000). North Carolina is now second to Iowa in hog production, however was initially fifteenth in the country between the 1980s–1990s. Hogs were initially evenly dispersed throughout the state prior to the 1980s, however, industrialization of hog production succeeded initial operations and monopolized rural locales and traditional farming practices (Hillard 1969; Pew Commission on Industrial Farm Animal Production 2008). As a result of increased production, the habitat for thousands of hogs were in Concentrated Animal Feeding Operations (CAFO's) which resembled factory facilities in the eastern part of the state where slaves once occupied (Nicole 2013). The challenges with Industrialized pork production with pungent odors released from hog manure that at times, penetrated inside of the homes of rural residents who lived near these facilities

(Nicole 2013; Kelly-Reif and Wing 2016; Wing 2000). The smell was so repulsive that local residents had to cover their noses while in their own homes. The dew from the manure often sprinkled on their cars, homes and outdoor laundry clothes lines.

CAFO's currently use hog waste for crops or as a spray on Bermuda grass. However, the odorous wastes contains toxic materials such as hydrogen sulfide and ammonia which researchers found led to eye irritation, respiratory problems, diminished quality of life and high blood pressure as a result of mental stress in local residents. Hog manure interfered with gardening and home visitors. In addition, antibiotic resistant bacteria strains occurred during hop operations and resulted in infections in workers, neighboring communities and families. Rural communities were mostly impacted by industrialized animal operating facilities. Current residents in the hog producing regions in North Carolina were predominantly rural minorities (Blacks, Hispanics and American Indians), experienced high poverty, low educational attainment, had inadequate access to healthcare, high unemployment and lacked political power. These rural residents no longer benefitted from the industrialization of pork, which incited environmental injustice and environmental racism arguments towards the hog industry. CAFO's are a globalized operation and therefore, state politicians supported and protected the financial interests of the hog industry. State legislation (NC House Bill 405) protected the hog industry from disclosure of vital information to citizens, researchers and workers. Gag laws prevented any scrutiny or documentation of the industries' operations including working conditions, food safety, animal abuse or health impacts which further exploited rural environmental justice movements associated with classism, racism and imperialism.

SDH: Food Insecurity

The United States Department of Agriculture (2016) defined food security as having sufficient access to quality and affordable foods to achieve a healthy lifestyle. In 2016, food insecurity affected 12.3% of U.S. households. This rate decreased from 14.9% in 2014 and 12.7% in 2015. Rural areas shared the greatest burden of food insecurity in the U.S. Studies showed that approximately fourteen percent of the urban population struggled with food insecurity compared to fifteen percent of rural populations (Coleman-Jensen et al. 2017). The prevalence of food insufficiency is at 17% in the rural South, which is the highest in the nation followed by the rural west at 14%, rural Northeast at 12% and the Midwest at 12% (Gundersen et al. 2017). Additional research confirms that 67% of rural counties in America had food insecurity rates well above the national average.

Eight percent of households with children were impacted by food insecurity in 2016 (Coleman-Jensen et al. 2017). Low food security affected 7.2% of children and 0.8% of children experienced very low food security which indicated patterns of inconsistent, normal food intake interrupted periodically during 2016. Households with older children had higher rates of food insecurity. Food insecure impaired cognitive function in children 6–11 years old and toddlers (Alaimo et al. 2001;

Zaslow et al. 2009). U.S. Food insecure adolescents experienced mental health issues at higher rates than adolescents with stable food environments at 28.7 and 9.2%, respectively and emotional and conduct issues (Poole-Di Salvo et al. 2016). They also experienced difficulty with developing or maintaining friendships with peers, poorer health, more suspensions, chronic absenteeism, anxiety and substance abuse (Shanafelt et al. 2016; Alaimo et al. 2001; McLaughlin et al. 2012). Rural counties in the U.S. had the highest rates of food insecure children, at 86% compared to urban counties (Gundersen et al. 2017). Studies reported by Shanafelt et al. (2016) showed that rural adolescents who lived in unstable household food environments were less physically active, had lower grade point averages. Females reported their health status as less than optimal and had lower attendance than their food secure, male rural counterparts. Poverty was the strongest indicator that worsened food insecure environments in households with children, irrespective of geography and demographics (USDA 2016).

The unique expression of the social determinants of health in rural areas fosters challenges in food security including access to public transportation, concentrated poverty, unemployment, inadequate communication networks and education (Gundersen et al. 2017). Rural populations, especially in the South were challenged with adequate transportation services to access healthy grocery stores or food assistance programs. Studies from Campbell et al. (2017) and Piontak and Schulman (2014) showed that rural areas had a shortage of large food retailers, therefore, these populations relied on convenience stores which consisted of less healthy food options and higher prices. If large marketplaces were available in rural areas (i.e. Walmart), rural populations traveled longer distances to these grocers compared to their urban counterparts, which caused food deserts. In addition, farmers' markets and food assistance programs such as food pantries and soup kitchens were less prevalent in rural areas. Poverty was higher in rural southern states relative to the nation and 44% of women in the South had female, single headed households, compared to 32% in the suburbs. Unemployment and underemployment were persistent challenges in rural areas, especially since the economic downturns in 2008, which preceded food insecurity in rural households. Given the presence of spatial inequalities in food availability and the absence of adequate infrastructure, rural and remote regions persistently remained at a disadvantage to achieving food sufficiency compared to their urban counterparts.

SDH: Digital Technology

Rural Americans faced the largest disparity in digital inequality. Rural communities lacked the infrastructure to implement broadband access and with constrained resources for construction, deployment remained costly (Education SuperHighway 2017; Federal Communications Commission (FCC) 2016). According to the FCC (2016), 39% of rural Americans also lacked advanced technological capabilities compared to 4% Americans in urban communities. In addition, the cost for broadband connectivity for rural consumers was relatively higher compared to their urban counterparts due to low population density, which impacted supply and demand. Some evidence of this was demonstrated in a survey that showed rural Americans persistently lagged behind their urban counterparts in their usage of digital technology (Perrin 2017). Recent surveys showed a significant increase in home broadband access for rural Americans from 35% in 2007 to 63% in 2016. In spite of these advancements, the digital gap between rural populations and all U.S. adults is still at 10%. For example, rural Americans were less likely to use smartphones, computers, home broadband and tablets compared to urban and suburban Americans. Furthermore, the use of multiple digital devices was less likely among this group. In terms of online frequency, urban and suburban Americans reported greater usage at 80 and 76%, respectively, compared to rural populations at 58%. Rural populations with higher earnings utilized multiple digital devices at rates nearly comparable to their wealthier urban and suburban counterparts which indicated that lower income rural populations experience the greatest disparities in the use of digital technology (Carlson and Gross 2016). When race and ethnicity was considered, geographical differences remained unmitigated. Education attainment played an unfavorable role in disparities in digital technology usage for all rural residents except for college graduates where the rates were similar. The largest gap in the digital divide was among rural and urban populations with less than a high school diploma.

Internet access improved over the past decades in rural areas through government programs, however, rural businesses experienced some distress in technology usage, albeit articulated in digital marketing (Richmond et al. 2017). Prior studies from Pociask (2005) revealed that small rural businesses seldomly used broadband services. Such services were commonly used in businesses for website creation or social media purposes, both of which were instrumental in economic vitality, the capacity to target diverse and distant markets, expansive customer reach and communications. Additional studies showed evidence that the internet contributed to a growth in the U.S. Gross Domestic Product (du Rausas et al. 2011). Small enterprises lacked the capacity to compete with larger ones, especially through e-commerce (Abed et al. 2015). In Minnesota, 10% of small rural businesses compared to other regions utilized social media (Daun and Muessig 2012). In North Carolina, 22% of small rural businesses utilized facebook as a marketing strategy compared to 35% of their urban counterparts. In addition, 97% of urban businesses had established links to their websites from their facebook page compared to only 20% of rural businesses. In the absence of applicatory practices with internet technologies, the rural economy and job development is compromised and the overall rural-urban digital divide continues to remain staggered.

Digital inequality effected learning opportunities for children (Education Super-Highway 2017). According to the Federal Communications Commission (2016), 6.5 million children lacked access to the internet in U.S. public schools in 2017. Over 2000 schools still lacked broadband infrastructure and 77% of these schools were located in rural communities and small towns. Some of the barriers to internet access in education included pricing for digital infrastructure which was higher in certain school districts relative to others. Inadequate or non-existent internet availability impacted student completion of homework assignments (Meyer 2016). Affordability restricted students to internet access in their homes and they frequently accessed wifi signals in local establishments or in the library to complete assignments. Many researchers argued that students in rural and remote rural places were largely affected, however, suburban and urban students also experienced similar challenges.

Digital inequality also impacted efficient healthcare for rural Americans. Well documented in the scientific research, were transportation barriers for rural and remote residents, which limited access to timely healthcare. Rural residents traveled far distances to reach healthcare facilities. If specialized care was required at a local facility, air transportation served as an alternative measures for rural residents received needed healthcare services (Goodridge and Marciniuk 2016). With these daunting challenges rural and remote residents faced, telehealthcare ameliorated access the healthcare. Telehealth offered synchronous and asynchronous modalities for rural patients or patients with medical limitations to have live and distant communications with their physicians or medical staff through video conferencing and sharing information through images and texting (Toh et al. 2016). The deliberative outcome was feasible access to care, increased patient compliance, medication adherence and a stronger doctor-patient relationship.

Telehealth served as an amenable solution for rural residents to access care, however, these services were only plausible with appropriate infrastructure (Goodridge and Marciniuk 2016; Skoufalos et al. 2017). Users required adequate electricity and broadband connectivity and broadband connectivity was especially deficient in rural areas and in some instances, not affordable if maintenance and product updates were required. Users required up-front costs for equipment and technical support. Image sharing using videos required high bandwidth or resolution, all of which, were barriers to rural residents due to costs.

Public Health Solutions

While this chapter did not present a literature review on all of the SDH subscribed by the CDC and the WHO, a recurrent theme is threaded throughout the one's selected. The insufficient supply of the SDH in rural locales impedes opportunities for rural America to live a healthy lifestyle. For public health practitioners with a strategic focus to alleviate health disparities in rural populations, I present this model, rather strategy, to address the unmet social needs of rural populations:

Step 1: Identify the rural landscape of interest. A substantive identification of the landscape includes: demographics (race/ethnicity, gender, citizenship status, population density, etc.), farming/non-farming land use, environmental structures
Step 2: Identify a health issue(s) you want to target and research relevant health statistics (i.e. individual risk related behaviors, morbidity and mortality rates)
Step 3: Conduct a Social Determinants of Health Assessment. A practical assessment allows you to evaluate the quality and availability of the SDH in your select rural

community of interest. There are many tools available however, I recommend the Community Health Needs Assessment (CHNA), which is a toolkit widely used at the national and local levels in organizations, medical institutions, health departments, etc. The intent of the toolkit is to reduce health disparities and advance equity in the social determinants of health through an analysis of a communities' needs and assets (Community Commons, n.d.).

Step 4: Funding Research: Research government, non-profit grants available for the SDH(s) you want to address and APPLY

Step 5: Implementation. Once funding is received, and implementation is underway, continue to research other areas of funding to promote sustainability.

The public health strategy presented above is not meant to walk individual practitioners through intermittent steps for a specific SDH intervention, i.e. partnership development with local residents, stakeholders and businesses, community engagement, qualitative interviews with the community of interest, or grassroots mobilization action strategies. These strategies are well documented in the scientific literature and *implied*, in this intervention. Therefore, the goal is for practitioners to by-pass all other measures that proved to be non-sustainable and to use the starting point to address rural health disparities with a dialogue on the Social Determinants of Health and understanding the impact a lack of social determinants of health has on the rural landscape so that public health practitioners can dispatch needed resources for rural communities to overcome such challenges more swiftly.

References

Abed, S. S., Dwivedi, Y. K., & Williams, M. D. (2015). Social media as a bridge to e-commerce adoption in SMEs: A systematic literature review. *The Marketing Review, 15*(1), 39–57.

Alaimo, K., Olson, C. M., & Frongillo, E. A. (2001). Food insufficiency and American school-aged children's cognitive, academic, and psychosocial development. *Pediatrics, 108*(1), 44–53.

Allen, R., Burgess, S., Davidson, R., & Windmeijer, F. (2015). More reliable inference for the dissimilarity index of segregation. *The Econometrics Journal, 18*(1), 40–66. https://doi.org/10.1111/ectj.12039.

Campbell, E. A., Shapiro, M. J., Welsh, C., Bleich, S. N., Cobb, L. K., & Gittelsohn, J. (2017). Healthy food availability among food sources in rural Maryland Counties. *Journal of Hunger & Environmental Nutrition, 12*(3), 328–341. https://doi.org/10.1080/19320248.2017.1315328.

Carlson, E., & Goss, J. (2016). *The state of the urban/rural digital divide. National telecommunications and information* Administration, United States Department of Commerce. Retrieved from: https://www.ntia.doc.gov/blog/2016/state-urbanrural-digital-divide.

Centers for Disease Control and Prevention. (2014). Office of disease prevention and health promotion, *Social Determinants of Health*. Retrieved from: https://www.healthypeople.gov/2020/topics-objectives/topic/social-determinants-of-health.

Coleman-Jensen, A., Rabbitt, M., Gregory, C., & Singh, A. (2017). *Household food security in the United States in 2016, ERR-237, U.S.* Department of Agriculture, Economic Research Service. Retrieved from: https://www.ers.usda.gov/webdocs/publications/84973/err-237.pdf?v=42979.

Community Commons. (n.d.). *Community health needs assessment*. Retrieved from: https://assessment.communitycommons.org/CHNA/About.aspx.

Daun, T. R., & Muessig, H. (2012). Assessing the digital presence of rural Minnesota businesses: Basic methods & findings. In M. Vitcenda (Ed.), *Technical report, extension center for community vitality*. St. Paul, MN: University of Minnesota.

du Rausas, M. P., Manyika, J., Hazan, E., Bughin, J., Chui, M., & Said, R. (2011). *Internet matters: The net's sweeping impact on growth, jobs, and prosperity*. McKinsey Global Institute, p. 21.

EdBuild. (2018). *Fault lines: America's most segregated school district borders*. Retrieved from: https://edbuild.org/.

Education SuperHighway. (2017). 2017 *State of the states: Fulfilling our promise to America's students*. Retrieved from: https://s3-us-west-1.amazonaws.com/esh-sots-pdfs/educationsuperhighway_2017_state_of_the_states.pdf.

Federal Communications Commission. (2016). *2016 broadband progress report*. Retrieved from https://www.fcc.gov/reports-research/reports/broadband-progress-reports/2016-broadband-progress-report.

Gochfeld, M., & Burger, J. (2011). Disproportionate exposures in environmental justice and other populations: The importance of outliers. *American Journal of Public Health, 101*(Suppl 1), S53–S63. https://doi.org/10.2105/AJPH.2011.300121.

Goodridge, D., & Marciniuk, D. (2016). Rural and remote care: Overcoming the challenges of distance. *Chronic Respiratory Disease, 13*(2), 192–203. https://doi.org/10.1177/1479972316633414.

Greenhouse, L. (2007). *Justices limit the use of race in school plans for integration*. June 29, 2007. Retrieved from: https://www.nytimes.com/2007/06/29/washington/29scotus.html.

Gundersen, C., Dewey, A., Crumbaugh, A., Kato, M., & Engelhard, E. (2017). *Map the meal gap 2017: A Report on County and Congressional District Food Insecurity and County Food Cost in the United States in 2015*. USA: Feeding America.

Heflin, C., & Miller, K. (2011). *The geography of need: Identifying human services needs in rural America*. Rural Policy Research Institute. Retrieved from: http://www.rupri.org/Forms/HeflinMiller_GeogNeed_June2011.pdf.

Highsmith, A. R., & Erickson, A. T. (2015). Segregation as splitting, segregation as joining: Schools, housing, and the many modes of Jim Crow. *American Journal Of Education, 121*(4), 563–595.

Hillard, S. (1969). Pork in the ante-bellum south, a geography of self-sufficiency. *Annals of the Association of American Geographers, 59*, 461–480.

Institute of Medicine (US) Roundtable on Environmental Health Sciences, Research, and Medicine; Merchant, J., Coussens, C., Gilbert, D. (Eds.). (2006). *Rebuilding the unity of health and the environment in rural America: Workshop summary*. Washington (DC): National Academies Press (US). Retrieved from: https://www.ncbi.nlm.nih.gov/books/NBK56974/. (4. The built environment and health in rural areas).

Kelly-Reif, K., & Wing, S. (2016). Urban-rural exploitation. An underappreciated dimension of environmental injustice. *Journal of Rural Studies, 47*, 350–358.

Kuczewski, M. (2016). The really new Jim Crow: Why bioethicists must ally with undocumented immigrants. *American Journal of Bioethics, 16*, 21–23.

Logan, J. R., & Burdick-Will, J. (2017). School segregation and disparities in urban, suburban, and rural areas. *The Annals of the American Academy of Political and Social Science, 674*(1), 199–216. https://doi.org/10.1177/0002716217733936.

McLaughlin, K. A., Green, J. G., Alegria, M., Jane Costello, E., Gruber, M. J., Sampson, N. A., et al. (2012). Food insecurity and mental disorders in a national sample of U.S. adolescents. *Journal of the American Academy of Child and Adolescent Psychiatry, 51*, 1293–1303.

Meyer, L. (2016). Home connectivity and the homework gap. *THE Journal, 43*(4), 16.

Nicole, W. (2013). CAFOs and environmental justice: The case of North Carolina. *Environmental Health Perspectives, 121*(6), a182–a189. https://doi.org/10.1289/ehp.121-a182.

Perrin, A. (2017). *Digital gap between rural and nonrural America persists, pew research center*. Retrieved from: http://www.pewresearch.org/fact-tank/2017/05/19/digital-gap-between-rural-and-nonrural-america-persists/.

Pew Commission on Industrial Farm Animal Production. (2008). *Putting meat on the table: Industrial farm animal production in America.* (2008). Pew Charitable Trusts and Johns Hopkins Bloomberg School of Public Health.

Piontak, J., & Schulman, M. (2014). Food insecurity in rural America. *Contexts, 13,* 75–77.

Poole-Di Salvo, E., Silver, E. J., & Stein, R. K. (2016). Household food insecurity and mental health problems among adolescents: What Do Parents Report? *Academic Pediatrics, 16*(1), 90–96.

Pociask, S. (2005). Broadband use by rural small business. *SBA Small Business Research Summary, 269,* 1–34.

Richmond, W., Rader, S., & Lanier, C. (2017). The "digital divide" for rural small businesses. *Journal of Research in Marketing and Entrepreneurship, 19*(2), 94–104. Retrieved from https://csuglobal.idm.oclc.org/login?url; https://search-proquest-com.csuglobal.idm.oclc.org/docview/1973893019?accountid=38569.

Rural Health Information Hub. (2018). *Social determinants of health for rural people.* Retrieved from: https://www.ruralhealthinfo.org/topics/social-determinants-of-health#rural-difference.

Shanafelt, A., Hearst, M., Wang, Q., & Nanney, M. (Susie). (2016). Food insecurity and rural adolescent personal health, home and academic environments. *The Journal of School Health, 86*(6), 472–480. http://doi.org/10.1111/josh.12397.

Skoufalos, A., Clarke, J. L., Ellis, D. R., Shepard, V. L., & Rula, E. Y. (2017). Rural aging in America: Proceedings of the 2017 connectivity summit. *Population Health Management, 20*(Suppl 2), S-1–S-10. http://doi.org/10.1089/pop.2017.0177.

Solari, C. D. (2012). Affluent neighborhood persistence and change in U.S. Cities. *City & Community, 11*(4), 370–388. http://doi.org/10.1111/j.1540-6040.2012.01422.x.

Strosnider, H., Kennedy, C., Monti, M., Yip, F. (2017). Rural and urban differences in air quality, 2008–2012, and community drinking water quality, 2010–2015—United States. *MMWR Surveillance Summary, 66*(SS-13), 1–10. http://dx.doi.org/10.15585/mmwr.ss6613a1.

Taylor, M. M. (2018). *Application of the Political Economy to Rural Health Disparities.* Springer International Publishing.

The Brookings Institution. (2018). *Growing economic segregation among school districts and schools.* Retrieved from: https://www.brookings.edu/blog/brown-center-chalkboard/2015/09/10/growing-economic-segregation-among-school-districts-and-schools/.

Toh, N., Pawlovich, J., & Grzybowski, S. (2016). Telehealth and patient-doctor relationships in rural and remote communities. *Canadian Family Physician, 62*(12), 961–963.

U.S. Department of Agriculture, Economic Research Service. (2016). Rural America at a glance: 2016 edition. (Economic Information Bulletin 162). Retrieved from: https://www.ers.usda.gov/webdocs/publications/80894/eib162.pdf?v=42684.

United States Department of Health and Human Services. Office of Disease Prevention and Health Promotion. (2018). *Social determinants of health.* Retrieved from: https://www.healthypeople.gov/2020/topics-objectives/topic/social-determinants-of-health.

Wing, S., et al. (2000). Environmental injustice in North Carolina's hog industry. *Environ Health Perspectives, 108*(3), 225–231.

World Health Organization. (2008). *Commission on the Social Determinants of Health. Closing the gap in a generation: Health equity through action on the social determinants of health. Final Report of the Commission on Social Determinants of Health.* World Health Organization: Geneva. Retrieved from: http://apps.who.int/iris/bitstream/handle/10665/43943/9789241563703_eng.pdf;jsessionid=E125050FA866C2C6DB529753B0ACEA91?sequence=1.

World Health Organization. (2018). *Health impact assessment: Social determinants of health.* Retrieved from: http://www.who.int/hia/evidence/doh/en/index5.html.

Young, R. (2015). Geographic distribution of acute chemical incidents—Hazardous substances emergency events surveillance, Nine States, 1999–2008. *Morbidity and Mortality Weekly Report, 64,* 32–38.

Zaslow, M., Bronte-Tinkew, J., Capps, R., Horowitz, A., Moore, K. A., & Weinstein, D. (2009). Food security during infancy: Implications for attachment and mental proficiency in toddlerhood. *Maternal and Child Health Journal, 13,* 66–80.

Chapter 4
Rural Health Disparities: The Policy Perspective

Political Will and Equity in Health Policies

Public health efforts to eliminate rural health disparities are futile in the absence of good governance (Malena 2009). Governance alone can facilitate or impede human development. A paucity of good governance cultivates poverty, political, social and economic ills, including social injustices. Good governance does not operate in silos, rather, it is participatory and citizens, organizations and governments coalesce to achieve transparency, equity and accountability in decision-making, especially for vulnerable populations. Participatory governance then proposes to empower and mobilize citizens to engage in a shared public process on social issues that directly impact their quality of life and well-being. However, participatory governance is incomprehensible without political will.

Political will is defined as, "the commitment of political leaders and bureaucrats to undertake actions to achieve a set of objectives and to sustain the costs of those actions over time" (Brinkerhoff 2000, p. 242). A lack of political will is the most common obstruction in the promotion of human development and a further hindrance on policy advancement for environmental protections, healthcare and economic reforms (Teitelbaum and Wilensky 2013; Blumenthal and Monroe 2009). According to Malena (2009), politicians exhibit political will in their actions to buttress participatory governance. Such actions are deliberative and demonstrative in the political actors' ability to engage in or create a platform for open dialogue with citizens that is not punitive, has the intent to advance equitable legislation, mainly in resource distribution, shows confidence in their capabilities to successfully embrace participatory governance principles and their capacity to bolster other key stakeholders. Finally, political will is also displayed in legislators when they exhibit a sense of urgency for social concerns which could entail a political, economic or social crisis that could result in high societal costs.

Lezine and Reed (2007) defined political will as, "society's commitment to support or alter prevention initiatives", (p. 2010). Society or government's commitment is what advances or impedes policies towards the sustainability of resources to build healthy communities. Collective actions on health equity and health promotion for

© The Author(s), under exclusive license to Springer Nature Switzerland AG 2019
M. M. Taylor, *Rural Health Disparities*, SpringerBriefs in Public Health,
https://doi.org/10.1007/978-3-030-11467-1_4

rural populations are inherently political and necessitates vested interests and collaborations (Zalmanovitch and Cohen 2015). Herein lies the gap between advocates who support health equity initiatives and policy practice. When scientific evidence substantiates the gross inequities in the social determinants of health in rural communities, the intent of decision makers and bureaucrats become more conspicuous. This prompts inquiries into the causal factors for persistent health disparities in rural areas and begs an analysis on the latter stakeholders. The absence or presence of political will remain central towards the advancement of resources to establish healthier rural communities. A greater understanding of what drives politicians towards policies to address this public health concern and under what conditions politicians lack motivation for a sufficient resolution, rather than remedial patchwork solutions (i.e. grants). This demands a knowledge of political preferences and elements that triggers politicians to act on an issue. If governments' have a predisposition towards distributive justice in health this would essentially prompt policies grounded in equity and perhaps, rural health disparities would not be as pervasive. The government's capacity to collaborate across different agencies to increase access to the SDH is one of many processes to address rural health disparities. However, the private intentions of bureaucrats, which often lack transparency to the public and decision makers, effects policy change as politicians demonstrate partiality towards bureaucrats over the public's interests. Market failures influence political decisions against the equitable allocation of public health goods and support the devolution of the welfare state under all economic circumstances. Social problems, such as health disparities, are considered a reflection of government failures and welfare policies to alleviate these problems often conflict with the economic interest of bureaucrats.

Given the challenges with the passage or implementation of sustainable and equitable public health policies (i.e. the ACA in the Trump political climate), theories on *health* political science emerged (Raphael 2014). Health political science centers on the term raw politics, which identifies public policy as a health determinant and gives recognition to the power structures that influence decision-making. Raphael (2014) claimed raw politics was a neglected domain, however, still largely responsible for the quality of and distribution of the SDH across race, class or gender. Raphael perceived any opposition to policies that support equity in the distribution of resources as a form of raw politics. For example, powerful interests shaped equitable public policies that had the potential to skew access to the SDH for vulnerable communities.

Some nations inherently support equitable health policies which created the climate for distributive justice for its citizens. Other nations, such as the U.S., U.K. or Canada ascribed to liberalism which submitted to a capitalistic system and therefore, less amenable to the implementation of healthy public policies. There are three different sectors that shape public policy and the distribution of the SDH. This includes the business sector, organized labor, power and influence and civil society power and influence. The business sector supports legislation on lower taxes for the wealthy and opposes government resources for social benefits and social security (Menaham 2010). Organized labor advocates for equity in the distribution of the SDH and more taxes on the wealthy. Trade unions underpin the strength of this sector. Civil society gains its power from public opinion, non-governmental institutions and agencies.

Essentially, healthy public policies support health with resources for populations to improve health, ensure access to the SDH, improve quality of life and divert elements that could harm health. However, in Social Democratic societies, equality in public policymaking is the primary ideological discourse and in liberal societies, the marketplace serves as the primary economic institution.

Decades of research proved that political will towards access to social goods is reached through pressure from community organizing efforts from affected citizens and civil society organizations (Ceukelaire et al. 2011). Mobilized efforts through social movements precipitated critical structural changes in government. Community organizations and trade unions established health protections for women and children in Cuba during the Soviet Union collapse. To resolve some of the conflicts between social classes, European trade unions repudiated child labor and secured universal health care. Abnormalities in the prevalence of respiratory problems in an area in Belgium sparked community mobilization efforts to petition against factories responsible for environmental pollutants which consequently led to the relocation of schools located near these factories. In the U.S., women's rights, civil rights and environmental regulations resulted from organized individuals, purposeful actors and organizations (Institute of Medicine 2014). These examples prove evidentiary that political will can entail a bottom up process such that individuals are empowered to advocate for their own rights and elicit political will to prompt policy changes.

Policy Approaches

Policy Logic Model for Rural Communities

Logic models are used as a planning tool for program design, program evaluation, program management and implementation (Hayes et al. 2011 and Das et al. 2014). Logic models are graphical representations of the goals of a program and identifies the resources, activities and results of a proposed program or project. The logic model makes theoretical assumptions about short and long-term outcomes. As a planning tool, logic models guide strategic decision-making, fosters critical thinking, communicates outcomes and makes predictions on the availability or potential challenges with resources that could impact a project. Evaluators use logic models to determine the impact of a program or to assess the process of implementation. For program management purposes, logic models represent a step by step approach towards the execution of a program. The basic components of the logic model include *Inputs* (resources, technology, materials), *Activities* (change agents, such as events or proposed services to execute the intervention), *Outputs* (measures the efficacy of activities), *Outcomes* (changes in knowledge or behavior for the population of interest, i.e. organization, individual or community) and *Impact* (assessment of long term change). Each category in the logic model are linked by arrows which represent a series of "if", "then" relationships and imply: if the following activities are present, then the following outputs are expected or if these outputs are expected, then these outcomes will follow (Kellogg Foundation 2004).

Logic models have been applied in the policy lexicon to: (1) develop more effective policies using policy documents; and (2) explain the effects of how healthy public policies address a public health problem (Wallis 2010, National Collaborating Centre for Healthy Public Policies 2013; Bauman et al. 2014). For the purposes of this chapter the latter policy logic model (PLM) structure is emphasized to construct a model to eliminate rural health disparities. Beforehand, some discourse of the former is relevant. Logic models were used in the context of policy documents to determine the most effective outcomes of a policy decision. As a policy document, the actors, stakeholders, policy researchers and alternative policy solutions are integrated in the PLM to represent the constructs of public policy making. These constructs include problem identification, political factors, political relationships and policy analysis. These type of policy logic models were instrumental in drawing comparisons between two policy options for a particular social problem. Legislators used this version of the PLM to adjudicate which policies to adopt, implement or to decipher which policies would render more effectiveness.

The PLM was also used to predict the outcome of a policy action or inaction. The prediction of a potential outcome was based on how a social problem is perceived. Immigration represents an example. Legislators can construct policy logic models on immigration reform based on two outcomes: (1) perceive immigration as a problem for society or (2) immigrants being an economic contribution to society. Neverthe-less, assumptions on outcomes constructed in the PLM require research evidence to establish validity for a specific political position, to mitigate ambiguity or to finance social programs (Langer et al. 2011). In the PLM, the arrows represent the research evidence that links each of the components of the logic model. Figure 4.1 is an illus-tration of a proposed policy logic model using policy documents on an environmental issue: Unconventional gas drilling, which affects many rural areas in the U.S.:

Policy documents (Inputs) are used in Fig. 4.1 to determine the efficacy of two policy decisions on unconventional gas drilling in rural areas, that is to approve or disapprove legislation. Each letter in the arrows (A, B, C and D) in the PLM represents the research evidence linking each category in the logic model:

A= represents research evidence for policy actions (Activities) to permit or not support unconventional gas drilling.

- McGlade, C., Speirs, J. and Sorrell, S. (2013). Unconventional Gas—A Review of Regional and Global Resource Estimates. Energy, 55(15):571–584
- Brown, J.P. 2014. *"Production of Natural Gas from Shale in Local Economies: A Resource Blessing or Curse?" Economic Review, Federal Reserve Bank of Kansas City* **99**(1): 119–147.

B= represents research evidence documenting the benefits and harm for uncon-ventional gas drilling in rural areas:

- Chen, H. and Carter, K. (2017). Characterization of the Chemicals Used in Hydraulic Fracturing Fluids for Wells Located in the Marcellus Shale Play. Journal of Environmental Management, 200:312–324.

Unconventional Gas Drilling

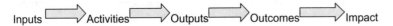

Inputs ⟹ Activities ⟹ Outputs ⟹ Outcomes ⟹ Impact

Inputs	A	Activities	B	Outputs	C	Outcome	D	Impact
Invited public Comments		**Do not permit** **Unconventional** **Gas drilling**		Less environmental damage to rural Landscape/less Exposure to toxins		Protect environ rights of rural populations		Environmental justice
Educational Materials from Industry				Acknowledgement of citizen opinions		Increase civic participation		Establish participatory governance for Rural commun
Educational Materials from Advocacy Groups						Less industry domination		Political empowerment
		Permit **Unconventional** **Gas drilling**		U.S. reliance on natural gas		Landowners; States benefit economically		U.S. recognition as an energy exporter
								Multi-billion Dollar benefit For industries
				Reduction in Common pollutants		Cleaner air		Alleviate climate change

Fig. 4.1 Policy logic model to address rural health disparities: environment concerns: Unconventional Gas Drilling

- W.L. Ellsworth. Injection-induced earthquakes. Science, 341 (2013), pp. 142–149
- J. Cooper, L. Stamford, A. Azapagic. (2016). Shale gas: a review of the economic, environmental, and social sustainability. Energy Technol, 4:772–792.
- Powers, M., Saberi, P., Pepino, R., Strupp, E., Bugos, E., & Cannuscio, C. (2015). Popular Epidemiology and 'Fracking': Citizens' Concerns Regarding the Economic, Environmental, Health and Social Impacts of Unconventional Natural Gas Drilling Operations. *Journal Of Community Health*, *40*(3), 534–541. https://doi.org/10.1007/s10900-014-9968-x
- Considine, T.J. Watson, R. and Blumsack, S. 2011. *"The Pennsylvania Marcellus Natural Gas Industry: Status, Economic Impacts, and Future Potential."* Department of Energy, Environmental, and Mineral Economics, Pennsylvania State University, University Park.
- Cooper, J., Stamford, L., Azapagic, A. (2016). Shale gas: a review of the economic, environmental, and social sustainability. Energy Technol, 4:772–792.
- J.A. de Gouw, D.D. Parrish, G.J. Frost, M. Trainer Reduced emissions of CO_2, NO_x, and SO_2 from U.S. power plants owing to switch from coal to natural gas with combined cycle technology. (2014). Earth's Future, 2:75–82

C= Represents the results (outcomes) of each of the proposed policy actions on unconventional gas drilling.

- Cotton, M. (2017). Fair fracking? Ethics and environmental justice in United Kingdom shale gas policy and planning. Local Environ, 22(2):185–202
- Malin, S. (2014). "There's no real choice but to sign: neoliberalization and normalization of hydraulic fracturing on Pennsylvania farmland," Journal of Environmental Studies and Sciences, Springer; Association of Environmental Studies and Sciences, 4(1):17–27.
- Hardy, K. and Kelsey, T. (2015). Local Income Related to Marcellus Shale Activity in Pennsylvania. Community Development, 46(4):329–340.
- Considine, T.J. Watson, R. and Blumsack, S. 2011. *"The Pennsylvania Marcellus Natural Gas Industry: Status, Economic Impacts, and Future Potential."* Department of Energy, Environmental, and Mineral Economics, Pennsylvania State University, University Park.

D= is the scientific literature review which represents the overall impact for each outcome in the PLM.

- Clough, E. (2018). Environmental justice and fracking: A review. Current Opinion in Environmental Science & Health, 2:14–18.
- Simonelli, J. (2014). Home rule and natural gas development in New York: civil fracking rights. Journal of Political Ecology, 21:258–278
- Minh-Thong, L. (2018). An assessment of the potential for the development of the shale gas industry in countries outside of North America. *Heliyon*, *4*(2), e00516.

The most successful logic models using policy documents occurs when stakeholders have clarity on the nature of the issue seeking policy resolution (Wallis 2010). One of the most salient limitations in using this version of the PLM is a

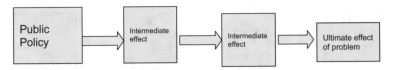

Fig. 4.2 Generic Policy logic model for planning healthy public policies (National Collaborating Center for Healthy Public Policies 2013)

lack of accountability for external influences which, at times, conflict with political decision-making. Also, these models were most useful in comparisons of only two types of policy options as illustrated in Fig. 4.1. Using policy logic modeling in this context is perceived as a micro approach to the more macro level approaches to understanding the policymaking process manifested through renowned theorists such as Paul Sabatier or John Kingdon (Sabatier 1993; Kingdon 2013).

The PLM can also be used to identify a public health problem and intersecting that problem with a healthy public policy (Morestin et al. 2010; NCCHPP 2013). Illustrated in Fig. 4.2, the PLM in this context is focused more on the intermediate effects the policy is expected to have upon implementation, to resolve a social problem, therefore, assumptions are made to determine the validity of the policy. This utility of the PLM represents a different scenario than the aforementioned concept which applied to policy adoption. These intermediate effects are logical assumptions and are not absolute. The effects are additive, such that when the process of policy implementation occurs, this prompts an initial intermediate effect, and then is expected to produce another effect, causing a chain of effects that sequentially impact the intended outcome of the policy, that is, to fix the public health problem. In this version, the PLM can be simplistic, exhaustive or comprehensive and include external factors or unintended consequences which can facilitate or counter the intermediate effects and subsequently the intended outcome.

The PLM for planning healthy public policies identifies potential weaknesses in the policy and promotes the development of solutions to address such weaknesses. This version of the PLM can also lead to the construction of a new PLM that has a more robust policy outcome. This process helps to establish validity in the chain of intermediate effects to ultimately decipher if the public health outcome associated with the policy is plausible. The PLM for healthy public policy guides data collection on the effectiveness and applicability of a policy to a specified public health problem. Scientific evidence that includes effectiveness data substantiates the chain of intended effects in the PLM. The visual representation of the causal chain between the policy and its effectiveness to address the public health outcome is more succinct than assessing numerous written documents. Each box between the policy of interest and the public health outcome guides the changes expected to occur that lead to the ultimate outcome. These changes should indicate an increase, decrease or alleviation of the intended effect. The number of effects in the PLM is not definitive and multiple pathways can be constructed in the model that lead to the ultimate outcome.

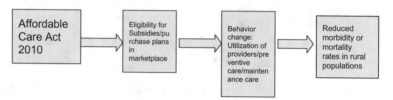

Fig. 4.3 Visual representation of the Policy Logic Model for healthy public policies to address rural health disparities: the PLM depicts the relationship between the Affordable Care Act of 2010 and the potential health-related outcomes: reduced morbidity and mortality rates in rural populations

Figure 4.3 establishes a planning tool and f ramework to evaluate the intermediate effects that occur after the implementation of a healthy public policy, for example the Affordable Care Act. It is worth noting that healthy public policies originate from community concerns, policy research, health impact assessments, existing or non-existing policies associated with the issue and the political climate (Bauman et al. 2014). The initial intermediate steps in this PLM includes policy implementation, which is the identification of the agency that administers the provisions of the ACA and community engagement, that is, ensuring the targeted community has access to program subsidies and providers. Each intermediate effect in the PLM requires its own evaluation of outcomes. For example, potential measurements can include the costs and benefits of using subsidies, if the program was delivered according to the provisions outlined in the ACA and health related behavior changes in the targeted population, which could ultimately lead to improved morbidity and mortality rates in rural populations. An evaluation of the intermediate effects can include various research methods such as qualitative methods community or stakeholders interviews, focus groups or quantitative methods.

Health in All Policies Approach for Rural Communities

The SDH informs us that the social and physical environment predicts health and life expectancy. To establish healthy communities through policy making, health officials coined the term, a "health in all policies approach (HiAP)," which encompasses all factors that predetermine health outcomes and not merely accountability to medical institutions (Wernham and Teutsch 2015). The HiAP approach is recognized nationally and globally by the World Health Organization, the Centers for Disease Control and Prevention and the European Union (Gakh 2015). HiAP incorporates the SDH in social policies and gives credence to the influence of non-health sectors, such as corporatism and quality of life measures. Non-health sectors also include some of the SDH, i.e. transportation, agriculture, housing, education and employment. Policies that focus only on access to health care are absent of other critical elements in the built environment that directly or indirectly influence healthy conditions for individuals to live, work, play and age (Wernham and Teutsch 2015). The HiAP approach warrants equity and a common public health agenda across all sectors and disciplines to improve quality of life and life expectancy. For example, a HiAP approach to asthma does not simply advocate for laws that provide access to treatment, but rather ensures that environmental and housing policies are formulated to eliminate toxins in the built environment or mold in housing structures that could aggravate this condition. In the rural landscape, a HiAP approach for residents afflicted with respiratory disorders considers chemical exposures in the water or air, adequate transportation, minimal proximal distances to the nearest hospitals and access to healthcare institutions and specialists with the capacity to treat these conditions.

The most widely used tool to influence decision-making using a HiAP for non health sector stakeholders was the Health Impact Assessment (HIA) which integrates any land use, energy, waste management, transportation and agriculture challenges. The HIA evaluates the impact of a specific plan, policy or program on a select population (Dannenberg 2016). HIA employs multiple data sources and methods on program effects and makes recommendations for best approaches to minimize such effects. HIA's consists of three different types of evaluation. The process evaluation focuses on HIA planning which includes preparation and research, impact evaluations which describes how the HIA impacted the outcome of decision-making and outcome evaluations examine any changes in population health or health determinants as a result of the HIA (Bhatia et al. 2014). Some limitations to HIA include a minimal structured method to perform a HIA, lack of resources and time constraints. In spite of these challenges, studies confirmed that HIAs directly impacted policy decisions on bicycle and housing plans and in some cases, enhanced community engagement, increased salience on public health concerns, advocacy skills that advanced the policy making process, enhanced collaborations between key stakeholders and decision makers and political will to consider HIA recommendations.

A HiAP approach is inherently systematic and involves a collaborative process to integrate public health into laws. Across all sectors, Governments, agencies, communities, the public and private sectors collaborate to establish an equitable landscape to advance population health (Gakh 2015; Wernham and Teutsch 2015). State laws have been structured towards a HiAP approach to facilitate (legally) sector and non-sector collaborations through boards, commissions and/or task forces. In California, the Governor executed an order to state agencies and Departments that all state business (transportation, environment and natural resources) operate with the intentions to improve and protect public health outcomes. At the county level, Knoxville, TN issued similar ordinances. Other state health department collaborated with health commissioners and their district boards of health to implement policies to safeguard consumer health and wellness. Another example, more nearer to environmental issues is rural landscapes is the case in Minnesota. Environmental toxins in wastes compromised clean air and water (Minnesota Executive Order No. 11–13 2011). The Governor's concern resulted in executive orders for state operations to use alternatively safe products to reduce air pollution and incorporate sustainability plans to evaluate progress to such goals.

A HiAP employs a range of tools to build healthier communities, establish agency accountability and to juxtapose public health practice and the legal system (Wernham and Teutsch 2015). Fundamental to a HiAP is community engagement and partnership development. Community engagement is cardinal to understanding areas of disenfranchisement and for the development of responsive policies that benefit community health and well-being. Partnership development between vulnerable communities and government, state or local agencies on public health concerns is a statement of conjecture for equity in the planning process for healthier communities. Partnerships with the private sector is also significant to a HiAP. Many private sector investments influence the SDH such as employment or pollution exposure, hence, strategic partnerships with public health agencies, communities and the private sector serves to collectively collaborate on minimizing health risks. However, the challenges with a HiAP is in establishing health imperialism in non-sector departments and communicating initiatives to stakeholders that excludes the traditional discourse on individual risk factors associated with diet or physical activity monitoring. In addition, the continuity of political will towards a HiAP remains a strong predictor for success and sustainability.

A HiAP calls for tools in the implementation science and a range of actors involved in the implementation process including public administrators, the public and private sectors and communities (Clavier 2016). HiAP establishes a new approach to policy making requiring implementing agencies to restructure how policy decisions are articulated and executed, which in turn, impacts a range of stakeholders directly affected by the policy. Public administrators have to possess the knowledge and capabilities to re-interpret policies based on what policymakers intended and also consider other sectors such as public health researchers and policy theorists to effectively understand how to integrate public health practice during policy implementation.

Concluding Remarks for Policy Models for Rural Health Disparities

From the perspective of rural health, distinguishing the need for *rural* SDH should be distinctive such that transportation agencies can articulate sustainable plans unique to rural versus urban residents. Infrastructure for roads and safer highways and sidewalks for the disabled and remote residents improves quality of life. In addition, a HiAP approach seeks recognition of corporate influence in decision-making in various industries, for example food products and recognize its effects on the farming industry and food security for farmers. Decision making on unconventional drilling in rural landscapes, from a HiAP, regards the precautionary principle, to prevent adverse health effects on rural communities and further holds the oil and energy industry accountable for any harmful effects incurred on rural residents due to drilling.

As these serve as examples of an approach to rural health disparities from the lens of public policy, the lack of political will to nurture participatory governance on a range of social issues that negatively impact rural populations demonstrates a devolution of local agency, retrenchment of social welfare policies which could potentially eliminate the disparity gap are masked with meager efforts to temporarily bandage the problems faced by rural Americans with sustainable or unsustainable funding, which is entirely dependent on the will of the existing political administration.

Rural health disparities can only get resolved through legitimate political analysis, research and action (Oliver 2006). Sustaining a healthy rural population benefits the economy, workforce and social organization. Ordinary citizens, including the poor, elderly and children, depend on the moral actions of local governments to ensure protections needed for survival and well-being. Governments (both local and global) have attained unanimity on the breadth of rural health disparities, however, similar to other public health issues that have gained heightened attention from policymakers, incremental policy change permeates the discourse when comprehensive and multidisciplinary policy efforts are eminent to the restoration of rural America. Consequently, political systems influence incrementalism and political history (and theory) informs us that the robustness and effectiveness of health policies at the global, national, state and local levels are measured according to various factors such as the degree of income inequality, industry regulations, political will, fiscal constraints, federal support, individual behaviors, corporatism and interest groups with the latter two factors being most common antecedents to incrementalism or policy inaction.

References

Bauman, A., King, L., & Nutbeam, D. (2014). Rethinking the evaluation and measurement of health in all policies. *Health Promotion International, 29*(1), 143–151.

Bhatia, R., Farhang, L., Heller, J., Lee, M., Orenstein, M., & Richardson, M., et al. (2014). *Minimum elements and practice standards for health impact assessment*. Retrieved from: http://advance. captus.com/planning/hia2xx/pdf/Minimum%20Elements%20and%20Practice%20Standards% 20for%20HIA%203.0.pdf.

Blumenthal, D., & Monroe, J. A. (2009). *The heart of power: health and politics in the Oval Office*. Berkeley and Los Angeles, California: University of California Press.

Brinkerhoff, D. W. (2000). Assessing political will for anti-corruption efforts: An analytic framework. *Public Administration and Development, 20*(3), 239–252.

Ceukelaire, W., De Vos, P., & Criel, B. (2011). Political will for better health, a bottom up process. *Tropical Medicine & International Health, 16*(9), 1185–1189.

Clavier, C. (2016). Implementing health in all policies—Time and ideas matter tool: Comment on "Understanding the role of public administration in implementing action on the social determinants of health and health inequities". *International Journal of Health Policy and Management, 5*(10), 609–610. http://doi.org/10.15171/ijhpm.2016.81.

Dannenberg, A. L. (2016). Effectiveness of health impact assessments: A synthesis of data from five impact evaluation reports. *Preventing Chronic Disease, 13,* E84. https://doi.org/10.5888/ pcd13.150559.

Das, B. M., Petruzzello, S. J., & Ryan, K. E. (2014). Development of a logic model for a physical activity-based employee wellness program for mass transit workers. *Preventing Chronic Disease, 11,* E123. https://doi.org/10.5888/pcd11.140124.

Gakh, M. (2015). Law, the health in all policies approach, and cross-sector collaboration. *Public Health Reports, 130*(1), 96–100.

Hayes, H., Parchman, M. L., & Howard, R. (2011). A logic model framework for evaluation and planning in a primary care practice-based research network (PBRN). *Journal of the American Board of Family Medicine, 24*(5), 576–582. https://doi.org/10.3122/jabfm.2011.05.110043.

Institute of Medicine. (2014). Roundtable on Population Health Improvement; Roundtable on the Promotion of Health Equity and the Elimination of Health Disparities; Board on Population Health and Public Health Practice. *Supporting a movement for health and health equity: Lessons from social movements: Workshop summary.* Washington (DC): National Academies Press (US); December 3, 2014. 2. Lessons from social movements. Retrieved from https://www.ncbi.nlm.nih.gov/books/NBK268722/.

Kellogg Foundation. (2004). *Logic model development guide: Using logic models to bring together planning, evaluation, and action.* Battle Creek, MI: W.K. Kellogg Foundation.

Kingdon, J. (2013). *Agendas, alternatives, and public policies.* Update edition, with an Epilogue on Health Care: Pearson International Edition.

Langer, E. M., Gifford, A. L., & Chan, K. (2011). Comparative logic modeling for policy analysis: The case of HIV testing policy change at the department of Veterans affairs. *Health Services Research, 46*(5), 1628–1645. https://doi.org/10.1111/j.1475-6773.2011.01283.x.

Lezine, D., & Reed, G. (2007). Political will: A bridge between public health knowledge and action. *American Journal of Public Health, 97*(11), 2010–2013.

Malena, C. (2009). *From political won't to political will.* Sterling, VA: Kumarian Press.

Menahem, G. (2010). *How can the decommodified security ratio assess social protection systems?* LIS working paper no. 529. Syracuse: Luxembourg Income Study.

Minn. Exec. Order No. 11–13 (April 8, 2011).

Morestin, F., Gauvin, F.-P., Hogue, M.-C., & Benoit, F. (2010). *Method for synthesizing knowledge about public policies.* Montréal: National Collaborating Centre for Healthy Public Policy. Retrieved from: http://www.ncchpp.ca/172/publications.ccnpps?id_article=536.

National Collaborating Center for Healthy Public Policy. (2013). *Constructing a logic model for a healthy public policy: Why and how?* Retrieved from: http://www.ncchpp.ca/docs/LogicModeleLogique_En.pdf.

Oliver, T. (2006). The politics of public health policy. *Annual Review of Public Health, 27*(1), 195–233.

Raphael, D. (2014). Beyond policy analysis: The raw politics behind opposition to healthy public policy. *Health Promotion International, 30*(2):380–396.

Sabatier, J., & Jenkins-Smith, H. C. (1993). *Policy change and learning: An advocacy coalition approach.* Boulder, Colorado: Westview Press.

Teitelbaum, J., & Wilensky, S. (2013). *Essentials of health policy and law* (2nd ed.). Jones and Bartlett Learning: Burlington, MA.

Wallis, S. (2010). Toward the development of more robust policy models. *Integral Review, 6*(1), 153–177.

Wernham, A., & Teutsch, S. M. (2015). Health in all policies for big cities. *Journal of Public Health Management and Practice, 21*(Suppl 1), S56–S65. https://doi.org/10.1097/PHH.0000000000000130.

Zalmanovitch, Y., & Cohen, N. (2015). The pursuit of political will: Politicians motivation and health promotion. *The International Journal of Health Planning and Management, 30,* 31–44.

Chapter 5
Rural Health Disparities: The Planning Perspective

Defining planning theory and practice in its application to rural health disparities presents both a challenge and opportunity for this chapter. First, the literature is limited in scope on the articulation of planning theories or practice for rural landscapes. Urban planning monopolized the interest of academia and to some extent, the globalized world. The overwhelming concern for the exogenous influence of capitalism in urban cities acting as a constraint to the urban built environment overshadowed the opportunity for rural discourse (Foglesong 1987). The inproficiency of the market-based economy to adequately supply the resources to sustain urban cities (sewerage, housing, roads, parks, etc.) was evidence for the appeal to state intervention, adding further focus on urban concerns (Foglesong 1987).

The rural landscape was not completely overlooked or unaffected by planners (Dandekar and Hibbard 2016). The industrialization of agriculture and natural resources invoked problems to the countryside. Rural communities were disconnected from economic benefits typically acquired from commodity production. Economic vulnerability, dilapidated areas and wealth establishment constituted challenges in rural planning. Industrialization elicited attractive wages and precipitated population loss in rural locales. In response to industrialization, rural planners aimed to secure economic development and quality of life by supplying some basic commodities to urban cities, such as lumber, minerals, food and fibre. However, rapid global industrialization incited market integration, which intensified planning and developments' focus towards metropolitan areas, shadowing the significance of non-metropolitan areas. At the turn of the century and with greater knowledge of the ramifications of globalization, urban ruralization set in and interests in rural planning resurfaced to counter or fix issues of rural concerns which involved climate change, future energy, food security and the ecosystem. The urban landscape started to adopt a more ruralized culture with appearances of community gardens and farmers markets and began petitioning concerns for energy reduction and abandoned areas. Rural planners concentrated on self-sufficiency which meant alterations to the physical design of rural landscapes. Plans for the construction of both town and country aimed to increase green ways, sociability and to maintain industry presence for employment opportunities. Rural planning then evolved to a localized

© The Author(s), under exclusive license to Springer Nature Switzerland AG 2019
M. M. Taylor, *Rural Health Disparities*, SpringerBriefs in Public Health,
https://doi.org/10.1007/978-3-030-11467-1_5

initiative with the understanding that the state was closer to and more knowledgeable of the priorities of local communities. However, social-political views, top down approaches and exploitation raised doubts about the rationality of the state as the best instrument to guide rural planning and development.

Historically, the planning discipline emerged in response to social problems prompted by industrialization (Dandekar and Hibbard 2016). Public health reforms, crisis in urban cities, social movements and public and private partnerships caused planners to serve as the mediator or negotiator (Fainstein and DeFilippis 2016). Davidoff (2016) argues that planners are not mediators, rather, they act as advocates to protect the interests of marginalized groups confronted with institutionalized domination and often excluded from traditional city planning. Planning for cities and regions intersects politics as these very forces shape city and regional development and planning (Fainstein and DeFilippis 2016). Therefore, capitalism and theories of the political economy inform and constrain planning practices. Social divisions have primacy in planning projects and is an extant obstacle which consequently, dissatisfaction in the outcome of such projects for some stakeholders is nearly predictable. Politics is embedded in social divisions and precepts structural differentiation. Social fragmentation caused by class, gender, religion or racial/ethnic conflict is at the heart of politics in planning. As Young (1990, 2000) describes, implicit in the politics is not merely demands for distributive justice which includes provisions for the social determinants of health, but rather the broader social institutions that have power to restrict material goods. Young argues for the planning of public spaces to uphold the inclusion of diversity in opposition to the suppression of differences (Young 1990, 2000; Fainstein and DeFilippis 2016).

The scientific literature describes the planners goals are to achieve equity in the social and economic distribution of resources for disadvantaged communities to create justice for cities (Thomas 2016). Planning equity is further biased towards participatory decision-making, mainly to support the powerless and to resist institutions and policies that impede these approaches. From the lens of social justice, planners must be aware of all actors that influence and compete for self-interests versus the publics interest. However, in the face of powerful economic interests, achieving equity presents a challenge for planners. Therefore, it is inconsequential to make assumptions that all planners have the capacity to accomplish equality under these latter circumstances. Nevertheless, planners who represent disenfranchised populations are likely to be motivated to pursue social justice due to their sensitivity and community bonds in urban societies. Hence, the need for diversity in the planning profession.

To advance community development, planners must not only have diversity in the profession, but in a pluralistic society, they must possess the capability to balance and serve the interest of all aspects of the public which include the polity, organizations, policymakers or ordinary citizens (Davidoff 2016). The balance implied by Davidoff (2016) is between urban politics and a democratic urban government. Inclusivity is thematic in the planning process and authenticates ordinary citizens as insightful, well-informed, participatory and responsive and anything contrary to this, petitions a unitary planning process. In unitary planning, a single agency is assigned, for example the city planning commission, to strategize on behalf of developing communities and obscures the concept of a pluralist society. In unitarism, it is then inconceivable for planners to serve as advocates for a public or private agencies to submit proposals during the planning process that support or counters their clients views or the perspectives of disenfranchised individuals.

Rural Planning

The aforementioned literature on planning theory and practice emphasized urban planning. The rural landscape was essentially depicted as agricultural and centering on agricultural policy. However, the rural landscape has changed tremendously in the 1990s. While the global population is mostly urban, the rural landscape nearly doubled since the 1950s (Dandekar and Hibbard 2016). Industrialization also affected the rural landscape, particularly agriculture. In rural areas in London, outward migration depopulated rural spaces due to lack of employment or infrastructure (Gallent et al. 2008). However, inward migrant and countryside attracted retirees from urban to rural landscapes. The rural economy shifted from simply an agricultural focus to an economic globalized markets sparking the interest for spatial planning. Many if not all of these concepts are applicable to the rural landscape.

Rural planning references policies and programs for human and physical capital development and diversity in economic development (Dandekar 2015). Physical capital development constitutes the preservation of agriculture and natural resources in the rural landscape. Human capital development is centered on building infrastructure, the accessibility (and quality of) education, housing, human services, health, etc. More recently, the challenges in global rural planning converged with issues in urban communities. The reduction of income disparities between rural and urban populations and structuring a sustainable economy beyond agriculture enterprises broadened concerns in rural planning. Rural planning in second and third world countries mollified redistributive justice of rural assets as developed nations supported laissez-faire economics. Second world countries, such as China eventually embraced a globalized approach. Third world countries emphasized increased agricultural production in their planning efforts to enhance quality of life for disenfranchised, low income rural populations. Rural planning should incorporate adaptations to the new economy, that is, the service sector and the information industry stabilized in metropolitan areas (Dandekar 2015). In The U.S. the service oriented approach to rural planning embraces support for infrastructure, advancements in digital technology and equitable quality of services evident in urban areas for job trainings, entrepreneurship and social welfare provisions. Rural planning *accepts* the evolving vision of the countryside as a place of retreat from city pressures for affluent populations.

Theory

Planning, in practice, is a coordinated set of multiple activities which incorporates the publics interest and deliberations on land development where the precedent for social justice is not implausible (Fainstein 2016). Planning emphasizes democratization in deliberation and principles of participatory governance. No particular social groups has primacy in deliberation, which is the essence of communicative planning. Communicative planning favors discursive interactions with equal opportunities for individual expression. Theorists criticize communicative planning theory for its inadequacy to acknowledge the leverage of external influences which instigate the social construction of decisions and outcomes (Murray 2005). Democratic deliberations are compromised in the presence of actors with an implicit bias towards capitalist interest (Fainstein 2016). Capitalism produces economic inequality and under these conditions, the working class is subservient to hierarchies of power which in planning, impedes legitimate deliberations and hinders egalitarian outcomes.

Foucaults' work exposed power relations, perceptions of sovereignty and modes of objectification of individuals classified as subjects (Smart 2002). Foucault further added that, "power is neither given, nor exchanged, nor recovered, but rather exercised and that it only exists in action" (Gordan 1980). In turn and with explicit modalities of power in practice, at some conjecture, the *subject* becomes conscious of his place in relation to power. Using Foucauldian theory, conflicts in rural planning are transitionary. Rural planning continued in subordination to urban privilege. Researchers, policymakers, consultants and academics characterized rural spaces from an urban lens. Rural planning acted subservient to a top-down perspective where marginalization of local knowledge and intelligence obstructed participatory rural planning (Kothari 2001). Recognition of local citizens' perception of areas for improvement, visions for local and economic development and interpretations of strategies to advance population growth represented a democratic process dishonored through urban objectivity. Researchers believed micro level politics influenced participatory rural planning projects (Johansen and Chandler 2015). In micro level politics, Johansen and Chandler (2015) claimed there were mechanisms of power that guided rural development projects and restricted local participation.

Institutionalising knowledge and competencies, structuring criticism and undermining the objectives of others was the fabric for such mechanisms of power in rural planning and often resulted in unintentional outcomes. Institutionalising knowledge and competencies involves actors in the planning process who perceive their knowledge and roles as legitimate and thus their interchange is from the standpoint of an institutional framework as opposed to between individuals. Conflict arises when the interchange is between researcher or consultant with local citizens. For example, an academics approach to rural development and planning mirrors the academics perception of rural qualities which becomes their foundation for institutionalizing their practical knowledge versus an emphasis on local (rural) knowledge which could lead to conflict or unanticipated outcomes in local communities. This mechanism of power is also depicted in rural planning if academia or other actors involved in the process determine who engages and at what capacity. In this case, the actors establish a selection criteria for local participation in contrast to an open invitation for all citizens and typically local citizens active in associations were often selected.

In the second mechanism of power, structuring of criticism, urban actors with similar interests establish alliances and/or formulates non-flexible viewpoints on the direction of the project. With such incontestable perspectives, the projects outcome is already decided, but the process is executed within a participatory framework. Input and preferences from rural participants are legitimized and encouraged. However, the communitys spirit and resilience is not incorporated in the final decision making process and does not influence the projects results. To some degree, the undermining mechanism of power is implicit in the second mechanism when the objectives and extent of participation from local residents are restricted from some aspects of the planning process by urban actors. Local participants can, in turn, undermine consultants and researchers by consistently questioning their intentions which could complicate the planning process. The undermining mechanism also entails opposition on goals and objectives between researchers, architects or planners. In addition, in the structure of planning venues, such as public hearings, urban actors can create conflict between local participants to the point where they undermine one another objectives.

Approaches

Participatory rural appraisal (PRA) is a method widely used in rural planning as an intervention approach to development (Narayanasamy 2009; Mukherjee 2004). This methodology evolved during an era when interventionists utilized top-down strategies and conformed to a dominant agenda in rural development. Local knowledge was not appreciated or incorporated into planning efforts. The methods used in PRA was intended to ascertain knowledge on rural life and conditions and enable rural populations to analyze and plan for action. PRA exploded globally in the 1990s and applied Freirans theme of participation in development, employed a bottom up strategy, encouraged the presence of local people and gave rural populations complete control during the process throughout the life of the project. PRA embraces a reciprocity in learning capabilities and collective action, especially with disenfranchised persons. The planning projects for PRA originally focused on socioeconomic development and expanded to other fields including community based organizations, environment, health, education, agriculture and food and nutrition.

The techniques in PRA were derived from a variety of disciplines, however, the methodology expanded from Rapid Rural Appraisal (RRA). RRA started in Kenya and India in the 1970s. RRA was academically, popularized by the 1980s (Heaver 2001). RRA methods was executed by urban professionals who extracted information on local rural issues using large surveys, direct observations, or semi-structured interviews, group walks, ranking and scoring, all of which, generated controversial results. RRA was criticized for its extractive and dominant approach where urban professionals collected and analyzed data and developed plans in the absence of feedback from rural participants. PRA was noted for its more relaxed, flexible and participatory approach that aimed to learn from and with rural people while pursuing similar methods. PRA triangulated data to ensure accuracy and considered an improved version of RRA. Non-government and field organizations were the main users of PRA compared to Universities who utilized RRA. RRA had a methods oriented approach compared to PRA, which aimed to study, share and learn about rural behaviors and conditions. RRA users had control over information collected and pursued publications, plans and reports as PRA users purposed their research for sustainable development and action such that participants too, owned and had the ability to control and analyze information. PRA advanced RRA from simply extracting information from local residents to facilitating and empowering local residents towards sustainable action. RRA users executed the role as investigator. PRA users acted as learners and facilitators to rural people and local citizens had dominion over data interpretation and outcomes.

The methods used in PRA and RRA share some similarities. For example, both methods utilize secondary sources, key informants, transect walks and timelines in data collection. Participatory mapping is also utilized in both approaches, albeit more frequently in PRA. Participatory mapping was utilized to determine the role of environmental factors in HIV prevention for rural adolescents in Kenya (Green et al. 2016). Researchers created a game using a basic map of their community which consisted of various roads, streets and areas of interest to youths such as schools and community features. A team of adults participated in the development of the base map. Through focus group participation, adolescents identified locations with a negative and positive influences within the community that impacted their behaviors.

PRA was applied as a tool in health planning for the development of prevention programs. NGOs utilized PRA techniques to develop a health needs assessment for an impoverished rural community in Pakistan that lacked healthcare services (Mahmood et al. 2002). NGOs acted as facilitator in a series of focus groups where community members identified health problems they considered a priority. The goal was to determine which type of healthcare services were of greatest concern and inaccessible to the community. Additional qualitative interviews assessed provider-patient relationships and availability. Quantitative surveys provided statistical information on the prevalence of disease. Researchers concluded that PRA was a vital tool for health planning in rural communities. PRA assisted in the development of a community needs assessment and increased community engagement in health care concerns. In the rural Jazan region of Saudi Arabia, PRA techniques was also used to develop a community health needs assessment (Bani 2008). Academics established a relationship of trust with rural community members and employed surveys, focus groups and key informant interviews to understand the prevalence of chronic and infectious diseases, high risk behaviors, environmental conditions to develop cost effective intervention programs.

In Kenya, PRA was used to understand how rural communities identified children with disabilities and to consider programs for community rehabilitation (Gona et al. 2006). Using focus groups and social mapping techniques, perceptions of children with disabilities were established. The results showed that rural communities in Kenya classified disabled children as those with a physical impairment, activity and participation restriction. Perceptions on why children were considered disabled ranged from beliefs of witchcraft, punishments from God or because they were orphans.

In the U.S., PRA strategies were employed to identify challenges to prevent health related illnesses in Latinos farmworkers in Washington (Lam et al. 2013). Focus groups were conducted to analyze their behaviors and attitudes about hydration. The results showed that Latino farmworkers associated the desire to sweat for weight loss concerns, cooling drinks were not necessary after heat exposure, caffeinated energy drinks were essential to remain vigilant at work and some had concerns about chemical treatment in the water at their worksites. Researchers concluded health education programs on heat related illnesses was essential for this population. In addition, improvements and strategies for health promotion should target the workplace and society.

Concluding Remarks on Planning Goals for Rural Health Disparities

While Participatory Rural Appraisal promises community engagement and potentially better developmental outcomes, the concern in rural planning is the objectification of local residents in subordination to urban actors. Urban actors must demonstrate the capability to execute a participatory framework and further be amenable to diversification in the projects' outcome. The decline of the dominant agenda in planning and development raises rural visibility such that the outcomes and consequences are accepted by all actors and are beneficial to local inhabitants and not just external actors. However, the challenge continues to be in the legitimacy of urban actors to pursue a planning agenda intended to operate in the best interest of rural versus capitalist interests.

References

Bani, I. (2008). Health needs assessment. *Journal of family & community medicine, 15*(1), 13–20.
Dandekar, H. (2015). Rural planning: General. In *International encyclopedia of the social and behavioral sciences* (2nd ed., 20, 801).
Dandekar, H., & Hibbard, M. (2016). Rural issues in urban planning: Current trends and reflections. *International Planning Studies, 21*(2), 225–229.
Davidoff, P. (2016). Advocacy and pluralism in planning In S. S. Fainstein & J. DeFillippis (Eds.), *Readings in planning theory* (pp. 427–442). Malden, MA: Wiley, Blackwell Publishers Ltd.
Fainstein, S. S. (2016). Spatial justice and planning In S. S. Fainstein & J. DeFillippis (Eds.), *Readings in planning theory* (pp. 258–272). Malden, MA: Wiley, Blackwell Publishers Ltd.

Fainstein, S., & DeFillippis, J. (2016). *Readings in planning theory* (4th ed.). Malden, MA: Wiley, Blackwell Publishers Ltd.

Foglesong, R. E. (1987). Planning the capitalist city: The Colonial Era to the 1920s. *American Journal of Sociology, 93*(2), 457–459.

Gallent, N., Juntti, M., Kidd, S., & Shaw, D. (2008). *Introduction to rural planning.* New York, NY: Routledge.

Gona, J., Hartley, S., & Newton, C. (2006). Using participatory rural appraisal in the identification of children with disabilities in rural Kilifi Kenya. *Rural Remote Health, 6*(3), 533.

Gordon, C. (1980). Power/Knowledge. *Selected Interviews and Other Writings,*1972–1977. New York: Pantheon Books.

Green, E. P., Warren, V. R., Broverman, S., Ogwang, B., & Puffer, E. S. (2016). Participatory mapping in low-resource settings: Three novel methods used to engage Kenyan youth and other community members in community-based HIV prevention research. *Global public health, 11*(5–6), 583–599.

Heaver, R. (2001). Participatory rural appraisal: Potential applications in family planning, health and nutrition programs.

Johansen, P., & Chandler, T. (2015). Mechanisms of power in participatory rural planning. *Journal of Rural Studies, 40,* 12–20.

Kothari, U. (2001). Power, knowledge and social control in participatory development. *Participation: The new tyranny,* 139–152.

Lam, M., Krenz, J., Palmandez, P., Negrete, M., Perla, M., Murphy-Robinson, H., et al. (2013). Identification of barriers to the prevention and treatment of heat-related illness in Latino farmworkers using activity-oriented, participatory rural appraisal focus group methods. *BMC Public Health, 24*(13), 1004.

Mahmood, M., Khan K., Kadir, M., Ali, S., & Tunio, R. (2002). Utility of participatory rural appraisal for health needs assessment and planning. *Journal of Pakistan Medical Association.*

Mukherjee, A. (2004). *Participatory rural appraisal: Methods and applications in rural planning, essays in honour of robert chambers* (2nd ed.). New Delhi India: Concept Publishing Company.

Murray, D. (2005). A critical analysis of communicative rationality as a theoretical underpinning for collaborative approaches to integrated resource and environmental management. *Environments, 33.*

Narayanasamy, N. (2009). *Participatory rural appraisal : Principles, methods and application.* Los Angeles: Sage Publications Pvt. Ltd. Retrieved from https://sso.umuc.edu/cas/login?entityId=https://login.ezproxy.umuc.edu&entityId=https://login.ezproxy.umuc.edu&service=https://sso.umuc.edu:443/idp/Authn/Cas.

Smart, B. (2002). Chapter 3: Subjects of power, objects of knowledge. In *Michel Foucault (9780415285339)* (pp. 64–117). Taylor & Francis Ltd/Books. Retrieved from https://sso.umuc.edu/cas/login?entityId=https://login.ezproxy.umuc.edu&entityId=https://login.ezproxy.umuc.edu&service=https://sso.umuc.edu:443/idp/Authn/Cas.

Thomas, J. M. (2016). The minority-race planner in the quest for a just city In S. S. Fainstein & J. DeFillippis (Eds.), *Readings in planning theory* (pp. 461–463). Malden, MA: Wiley, Blackwell Publishers Ltd.

Young, I. M. (1990). *Justice and the politics of difference.* Princeton, N.J: Princeton University Press.

Young, I. M. (2000). *Inclusion and democracy.* New York, NY: Oxford University Press.

Chapter 6
Conclusion: A Progressive Vision

Globally and nationally, health outcomes for rural populations appear dismal. Inequalities in health widened, geographically, for decades, as race, ethnicity and socioeconomic status remained the spotlight for literary attention. The convergence of theory and interventions to address these matters failed to identify the magnitude of geographical differences in health. Income provisions, cultural sensitivity and behavior modifications materialized as solutions to the race, ethnic and income juxtaposition. However, upon further analysis, these same factors augmented geographical health disparities.

Each chapter in this book represents discrete interpretations and approaches to address rural health disparities. The focus on public health, planning and policy approaches was not meant to discredit the capability of other disciplines such as sociology, anthropology or psychology, (just to name a few). Rather, the goals for this book was to offer public health practitioners, policy analysts and planners broader, concrete and viable solutions to eradicate rural health disparities at the local, state, national and global levels. Each discipline presented in this book, including the chapter on environmental injustices, coalesced around politics, capitalism and distributive justice.

The preceding chapters elucidated theories, models and practical solutions for researchers, academia and students to explore beyond the scope of this book. This book was intended to foster a multidisciplinary approach for the implementation of programs, policies and sustainable plans to create equitable spaces, eliminate health disparities and diminish capitalistic influence in rural affairs.

© The Author(s), under exclusive license to Springer Nature Switzerland AG 2019   57
M. M. Taylor, *Rural Health Disparities*, SpringerBriefs in Public Health,
https://doi.org/10.1007/978-3-030-11467-1_6

Index

C
Cancer, 1, 2, 4, 9–11
Capitalism, 22, 49, 50, 52, 57

D
Democracy
Digital inequality, 30–32
Dissimilarity index, 26, 27

E
Economic deprivation, 1
Economic inequality, 27, 52
Environmental injustice, 17, 20, 29

F
Food insecurity, 5, 21, 26, 29, 30
Fracking technology, 18–20, 22

G
Globalization, 49

H
Health disparities, 1–3, 12, 25, 32, 33,
    38, 57
Health in all policies, 44–46
Health planning, 54
Health political science, 38
Healthy public policy, 43, 44
Heart disease, 2, 4, 5

I
Income inequality, 2, 3, 47
Industrialization, 28, 29, 49–51

L
Laissez-faire, 51

M
Mechanisms of power, 52

O
Opioid abuse, 7

P
Participatory governance, 21, 37, 46, 52
Participatory Rural Appraisal, 53, 55
Planners, 49–51, 53, 57
Planning, 22, 39, 42–46, 49–53, 55, 57
Policy analysis, 40
Policy analysts, 57
Policy documents, 40, 43
Policy logic models, 39–41, 43, 44
Political ecology, 17, 22, 42
Political will, 37–39, 45–47
Politics, 25, 38, 50, 52, 57
Precautionary principle, 21, 46
Public health, 2, 3, 6, 19, 22, 25, 26, 32, 33, 37,
    38, 40, 43–47, 50, 57
Public health practitioners, 25, 32, 33, 57
Public policy, 38, 40, 46

R
Racial segregation, 27
Rural health disparities, 3, 22, 25, 26, 33, 37,
    38, 40, 41, 44, 46, 47, 49, 55, 57
Rural landscape, 1, 4, 9, 12, 17, 18, 20, 22, 32,
    33, 45, 49, 51

© The Author(s), under exclusive license to Springer Nature Switzerland AG 2019
M. M. Taylor, *Rural Health Disparities*, SpringerBriefs in Public Health,
https://doi.org/10.1007/978-3-030-11467-1

Rural planning, 49–53, 55
Rural populations, 1–6, 8–10, 12, 17, 22, 25,
        26, 28–32, 38, 44, 47, 51, 53, 57
Rurality, 1, 4, 5, 9, 11, 28

S
Segregation, 2, 25–27
Social Determinants of Health, 2, 8, 25, 26,
        30, 32, 33, 38, 50
Spatial injustice, 1

Spatial justice, 20

T
Toxic exposures, 26, 28

U
Unconventional gas drilling, 19, 20, 40–42
Unintentional injuries, 2, 4, 6–8
Urban privilege, 52

Printed in the United States
By Bookmasters